Neonatology
at a Glance

Neonatology at a Glance

TOM LISSAUER, MB, BChir, FRCPCH
Consultant Neonatologist
Winnicott Baby Unit
St Mary's Hospital
London, UK

AVROY A. FANAROFF, MD, FRCPCH
Gertrude Lee Chandler Tucker Professor and Chair
Department of Pediatrics
Case Western Reserve University
Eliza Henry Barnes Chair of Neonatology
Physician in Chief
Rainbow Babies & Children's Hospital
Cleveland, Ohio, USA

Associate Editors

RICARDO J. RODRIGUEZ, MD
Associate Professor of Pediatrics
Case Western Reserve University
Attending Neonatologist
Rainbow Babies & Children's Hospital
Cleveland, Ohio, USA

MICHAEL WEINDLING, MD, FRCPCH
Professor of Perinatal Medicine
Liverpool Women's Hospital
Liverpool, UK

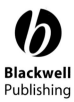

Blackwell
Publishing

First published 2006
3   2007

Library of Congress Cataloging-in-Publication Data

Neonatology at a glance / edited by Tom Lissauer, Avory A. Fanaroff.
   p. ; cm. — (At a glance)
  Includes index.
  ISBN 978-0-632-05597-5 (pbk. : alk. paper)
  1. Neonatology. 2. Neonatal intensive care. 3. Infants (Newborn)—Diseases.
  [DNLM: 1. Infant, Newborn. 2. Infant Care. 3. Infant, Newborn, Diseases—therapy. 4.
Neonatology—methods. WS 420 N4402 2006] I. Lissauer, Tom. II. Fanaroff, Avroy A. III. At a
glance series (Oxford, England)

RJ251.N22 2006
618.92'01—dc22

2005023987

ISBN 978-0-632-05597-5

A catalogue record for this title is available from the British Library

Set in 9.5 on 12 pt Times by Sparks, Oxford – www.sparks.co.uk
Printed and bound in India by Replika Press Pvt. Ltd

Commissioning Editor: Vicki Noyes and Martin Sugden
Editorial Assistant: Caroline Aders
Managing Editor: Geraldine Jeffers
Production Editor: Fiona Pattison
Production Controller: Kate Charman

For further information on Blackwell Publishing, visit our website:
www.blackwellpublishing.com

The publisher's policy is to use permanent paper from mills that operate a sustainable forestry policy,
and which has been manufactured from pulp processed using acid-free and elementary chlorine-
free practices. Furthermore, the publisher ensures that the text paper and cover board used have met
acceptable environmental accreditation standards.

Contents

Preface

This book provides a concise, illustrated overview of neonatal medicine. We have aimed to cover the breadth of neonatology in 89 double pages, with major topics confined to one or two double pages. This has been a challenging exercise as it would have been easier to write a longer book, but this format has forced us to identify the most important points and omit unnecessary details. The book has been designed to make learning easier and more enjoyable. Modern education emphasizes visual impact and this is reflected in this book. The layout, photographs and illustrations have been chosen to assist learning and make the book attractive and interesting. In addition, there are specific aids to learning, with boxes to highlight key points and questions and answers.

The book covers the preterm infant and the wide range of common or important neonatal clinical conditions and their management. It also puts neonatology into context, with sections on its history, epidemiology, perinatal medicine and a global overview, together with the care of the normal newborn and how to recognize the sick infant. The challenging topics of ethical issues, research, quality assurance, evidence-based medicine, when a baby dies, autopsy and neonatal outcome are also considered. Practical procedures are described, including neonatal resuscitation and neonatal transport; a description of cranial ultrasound and echocardiography have been included to inform the practicing clinician about them even if they do not perform these procedures themselves.

The book is written for pediatric interns and residents, medical students, neonatal nurse practitioners, neonatal nurses, therapists and midwives who care for newborn babies either on a neonatal unit or with their mothers in the normal newborn nursery (postnatal wards). Whilst the book describes the salient features of intensive care, such as stabilizing the sick infant and respiratory support, it is not a manual of neonatal intensive care, of which there are many.

The book has been a collaborative project between editors and contributors from both North America and the UK. Where practices differ between the two sides of the Atlantic this has been acknowledged and described. This collaboration has been highly educational and hugely enjoyable for the editors and contributors as well as improving the book by forcing us to concentrate on the principles of practice instead of the details.

We would like to acknowledge the help of many colleagues, in particular Drs Sunit Godambe, Maggie Meeks and Ezam Mat-Ali who contributed ideas and photographs whilst working on the Winnicott Baby Unit at St. Mary's Hospital in London, as well as Inga Warren, Consultant Therapist in Neonatal Developmental Care, who keeps the thoughts of neonatologists and neonatal nurses focussed on the baby and parents.

We would also like to thank our families for allowing us to spend so much time over several years on this project.

Tom Lissauer and Avroy A. Fanaroff (Editors)
Ricardo Rodriguez and Michael Weindling (Associate Editors)

Contributors

The editors are indebted to the following for their contributions to the chapters listed below:

Paula Bolton-Maggs
Consultant Paediatric Hematologist
Manchester Royal Infirmary
Manchester, UK
52 Anemia and polycythemia
54 Coagulation disorders

George Haycock
Professor of Paediatrics and Consultant Paediatric Nephrologist
Guy's Hospital
London, UK
48 Kidney and urinary tract disorders: antenatal diagnosis
49 Kidney and urinary tract disorders

Susan Izatt
Assistant Clinical Professor of Pediatrics
Duke University Medical Center
Durham, North Carolina, USA
12 Neonatal resuscitation

Helen Kingston
Consultant Geneticist
St Mary's Hospital
Manchester, UK
8 Birth defects and genetic disorders

Carolyn Lund
Neonatal Clinical Nurse Specialist
Children's Hospital
Oakland, California, USA
55 Skin

Hermione Lyall
Consultant in Paediatric Infectious Diseases
St Mary's Hospital
London, UK
10 Congenital infection
40 Neonatal infection
41 Specific bacterial infections
42 Viral infections

Neil McIntosh
Professor of Child Life & Health and Consultant Neonatologist
University of Edinburgh
Edinburgh, UK
65 Ethics
66 Research and consent

Patrick McNamara
Staff Neonatologist
Hospital for Sick Children
Toronto, Ontario, Canada
77 Echocardiography for the neonatologist

Maggie Meeks
Consultant Neonatologist
Leicester General Hospital
Leicester, UK
21 Common problems of term infants
73 Common practical procedures
74 Central venous catheters and intraosseous cannulation
75 Chest tubes and exchange transfusions

Michael Reed
Professor of Pediatrics
Case Western Reserve University School of Medicine
Rainbow Babies & Children's Hospital
Cleveland, Ohio, USA
61 Pain

Jonathan Stevens
Staff Neonatologist
Northern Alberta Neonatal Program
Edmonton, Alberta, Canada
71 Transport of the sick newborn infant

Eileen Stork
Associate Professor of Pediatrics
Case Western Reserve University School of Medicine
Rainbow Babies & Children's Hospital
Cleveland, Ohio, USA
59 Bone and joint disorders

Nim Subhedar
Consultant Neonatologist
Liverpool Women's Hospital
Liverpool, UK
25 Respiratory support
27 Lung development and surfactant
28 Respiratory distress syndrome

Dharmapuri Vidyasagar
Professor of Pediatrics
University of Illinois College of Medicine
Chicago, Illinois, USA
1 Milestones in neonatology

Inga Warren
Consultant Therapist in Neonatal Developmental Care
St Mary's Hospital
London, UK
23 Developmental care

Deanne Wilson-Costello
Associate Professor of Pediatrics
Case Western Reserve University School of Medicine
Rainbow Babies & Children's Hospital
Cleveland, Ohio, USA
37 Outcome of very low birthweight infants
69 Follow-up of high-risk infants

We would also like to thank Dr David Clark, Professor and Chairman, The Children's Hospital, Albany, New York, USA, and Dr Alan Spitzer, Senior Vice President and Director, The Center for Research and Education, Pediatrix Medical Group, Sunrise, Florida, USA, for contributing photographs and Dr Carlos Sivit, Professor of Radiology and Director of Pediatric Radiology, Rainbow Babies & Children's Hospital, Cleveland, Ohio, USA, for providing the cranial ultrasound photographs for Chapter 76.

The care of newborn infants has evolved over the last century from simple and empirical care to modern, evidence-based, high-tech medicine. Neonatal mortality has correspondingly declined dramatically from 40/1000 livebirths in 1900 to 4/1000 in 2003 in the US and UK. Improved obstetric care and maternal health and nutrition have also contributed. It was only in the 1950s that medical care of healthy and sick newborn infants was transferred from obstetricians to pediatricians. The specialty of neonatology developed only in the 1960s, and the first certifying examination for physicians in the US was held in 1975.

Incubators/thermal regulation

- 1890s: Tarnier in France showed that a warm, controlled environment reduced mortality of infants <2 kg from 66% to 38% (Fig. 1.1).
- 1893: Budin, Tarnier's student, established the first unit for premature babies in Paris, emphasizing thermal regulation and breast-feeding.
- Early 1900s: premature babies in incubators were exhibited in fairs around Europe and the US (Fig. 1.2).
- 1950s: Silverman in the US conducted elegant randomized controlled trials to confirm the beneficial effects of thermal control (including humidity) on mortality.

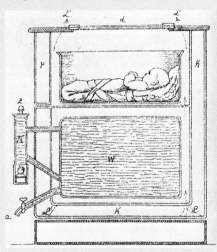

Fig. 1.1 The Tarnier incubator. The water was heated by the oil flame. The baby was kept warm by the heated air circulating around the incubator.

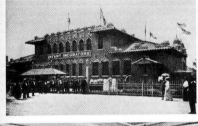

Fig. 1.2 Incubators with premature babies at the Pan-American Exposition, Buffalo, New York in 1901. (Source: Silverman WA. Incubator-baby side shows. *Pediatrics* 1979; **64**:127. Courtesy of the American Academy of Pediatrics.)

Nutrition

- 1880s: Tarnier and Budin recommend early feeding and intragastric 'gavage' feeding via a rubber tube.
- 1907: Rotch in US introduces infant formula. Breast-feeding declines as some believed formula was superior.
- 1940s: Gavage feeding via a nasogastric tube used in neonatal units.
- 1940s: Feeding of preterm infants delayed up to 4 days to avoid aspiration. Adverse effects (hypoglycemia, increased bilirubin and impaired development) recognized only in the 1960s, and early feeding reintroduced.
- 1960s: TPN (total parenteral nutrition) by central venous catheter introduced centrally, then via peripheral veins.
- 1960s: Infant formula associated with neonatal tetany from hypocalcemia and hemolysis from vitamin E deficiency.
- 1980s: Development of special formulas for very low birthweight infants.
- 1980s: Resurgence of use of breast milk. Human milk fortifiers developed for preterm infants.
- 2000s: Addition of long-chain polyunsaturated fatty acids (LCPUFA) to formula.

Antibiotics

Before antibiotics, mortality from neonatal sepsis was almost 100%, but it declined markedly when penicillin was introduced in 1944. The organisms causing sepsis have changed (Fig. 1.3).

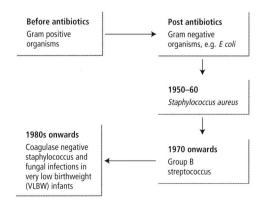

Fig. 1.3 Change with time of main organisms causing neonatal infection.

Rhesus hemolytic disease

Kernicterus, from bilirubin deposition in the brain from rhesus disease, was first described in 1938. Exchange transfusions became a common procedure in neonatal units and saved an estimated 8000 lives/year in the US alone. Rhesus disease is now almost completely prevented by prophylaxis.
• 1925: Hart describes first exchange transfusion – blood in via saphenous vein, out from anterior fontanel.

• 1940: Landsteiner discovers rhesus factor.
• 1945: Coomb develops Coomb's test (direct antiglobulin test, DAT) to detect rhesus agglutinins.
• 1947: Diamond describes exchange transfusion via umbilical vein with rubber catheter.
• 1963: Liley introduces intrauterine transfusion.
• 1964: Freda and Clarke develop prophylaxis with anti-D immunoglobulin.

Respiratory distress syndrome (RDS)

Oxygen therapy, monitoring and respiratory support
Whereas about 25 000 infants died every year in the US from RDS in the early 1950s, by 2003 there were fewer than 500 such deaths. This has resulted from:
• understanding the pathogenesis of RDS, which enabled development of surfactant replacement therapy
• antenatal corticosteroids to induce surfactant and lung maturation
• developments in respiratory support:
  – oxygen therapy
  – mechanical ventilators, first shown to improve survival by Swyer in Toronto and Reynolds in London (1965); continuous positive airway pressure (CPAP) introduced by Gregory
• ability to closely monitor vital signs and blood gases
  – cardiorespiratory monitors for neonates
  – measurement of blood gases on small blood samples
  – umbilical/peripheral artery catheters
  – transcutaneous arterial O_2 and CO_2 monitors
  – non-invasive oxygen saturation monitors.

History of respiratory distress syndrome (surfactant deficiency)
• 1955: Pattle describes properties of surfactant.
• 1956: Clements isolates surfactant.
• 1959: Avery and Mead demonstrate lack of surfactant in preterm lungs.
• 1972: Liggins and Howie – prenatal corticosteroids induce lung maturity.
• 1980: Fujiwara – first surfactant replacement therapy.
• 1985: Multicenter clinical trials of natural and artificial surfactant replacement therapy.
• 1989: Surfactant therapy approved.

Key point

For the last 50 years RDS has been the major focus of research in neonatology. Understanding its pathophysiology and the biochemistry of surfactant has been the key to developing surfactant replacement therapy and designing appropriate respiratory support, which have dramatically decreased mortality.

Development of neonatal intensive care

• 1922: First neonatal unit in US in Chicago by Hess; in UK by Crosse in Birmingham in 1945.
• 1960s and 1970s: Development of regional neonatal intensive care units with dedicated staff, introduction of CPAP and mechanical ventilation.
• 1970s: Ultrasound to identify intraventricular hemorrhage.
• 1970s: Ability to safely perform surgery in tiny infants.
• 1980s: Development of multicenter clinical trials, national and international.
• 1980s: ECMO (extracorporeal membrane oxygenation).
• 1990s: NO (nitric oxide) therapy for persistent pulmonary hypertension of the newborn.

Challenges for the future

• Reduce prematurity, hypoxic–ischemic brain injury, neonatal infection, congenital abnormalities.
• Avoid complications of preterm infants: brain injury, necrotizing enterocolitis, bronchopulmonary dysplasia (chronic lung disease), retinopathy of prematurity.
• Practice evidence-based medicine.
• Reduce iatrogenic disease, e.g. medication errors.
• Develop better non-invasive monitoring.
• Enhance nursery environment.
• Confront ethical dilemmas at the limit of viability.
• Improve and extend care at home of technology-dependent infants.

Epidemiology is the study of the causes of disease or death. In perinatology the focus is on the causes of illness and death in mothers, the fetus and newborn infants.

Definitions

Newborn infant
- *Preterm: <37 completed weeks of gestation.*
- *Term: 37–41 completed weeks of gestation.*
- *Post-term: ≥42 completed weeks of gestation.*
- *Low birthweight (LBW): <2500 g.*
- *Very low birthweight (VLBW): <1500 g.*
- *Extremely low birthweight (ELBW): <1000 g.*

Mortality
- *Maternal mortality: the number of maternal deaths (during pregnancy and within 42 days postpartum) per 100 000 live births.*
- *Stillbirth (fetal death): definition varies between countries and according to use – fetus born with no signs of life after 20 or 28 completed weeks or birthweight >350 g or ≥500 g in the US, fetus born with no signs of life after 24 weeks in the UK.*
- *Perinatal mortality rate (PMR): stillbirths plus early neonatal deaths (up to 6 completed days of life) per 1000 live and stillbirths.*
- *Neonatal mortality rate (NMR): deaths in the first 4 weeks (27 completed days) of life per 1000 live births.*
- *Post-neonatal mortality rate: deaths from 28 days until 1 year per 1000 live births.*
- *Infant mortality rate: deaths in the first year of life per 1000 live births.*

These indicators are valuable as measures of the health of a region or country and allow comparisons between them and monitoring of changes over time.

Births

There are 4 million births per year in the US and 700 000 in the UK. The average age of a mother giving birth has risen to 25 years in the US and to 29 years in the UK (average age at first child 27 years). There has been a steady rise in the birth rate for women in their thirties and forties.

Maternal mortality

The huge reduction in maternal mortality is one of the most dramatic improvements in health. In the US, maternal mortality declined from 582/100 000 live births in 1936 to 7/100 000 in 1999. This is due to reduced mortality from puerperal sepsis following the development of antibiotics, improved obstetric care, availability of blood and blood products, and better maternal health.

Perinatal mortality

The causes of perinatal mortality are shown in Fig. 2.1. The risk to the infant of perinatal death is almost 100 times that for the mother.

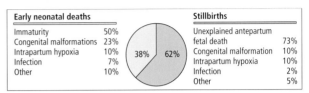

Fig. 2.1 Causes of perinatal mortality (England and Wales, 1998).

In the US, the perinatal mortality fell from 13/1000 live and stillbirths in 1980 to 6.9/1000 in 2002. The decline has occurred not only because of advances in neonatal care, but also from improved maternal health and nutrition and obstetric care.

Neonatal mortality

Neonatal mortality has declined steadily over the last 25 years (Fig. 2.2).

Birthweight is the main risk factor for neonatal mortality. The neonatal mortality rate is therefore largely determined by the birthweight distribution and birth weight-specific mortality rates (Table 2.1).

Table 2.1 Birthweight distribution and neonatal mortality (US, 2000).

Birthweight	Births (%)	Neonatal mortality rate (per 1000 live births in specified groups)
>2500 g	92.4	0.9
<2500 g	7.6	48
<1500 g	1.4	214

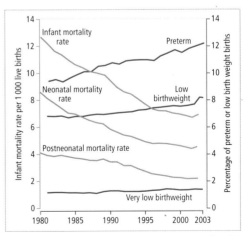

Fig. 2.2 Neonatal and infant mortality in the US have declined markedly since 1980. This is in spite of an increase in the proportion of infants born preterm or with low birth weight, mainly from the rise in maternal age and assisted reproduction. However, the proportion of very low birthweight (VLBW) infants has remained unchanged. (Source: Annual Summary of Vital Statistics – 2003. Martin JA *et al. Pediatrics* 2005; **115**: 619–634.)

EPICure Study

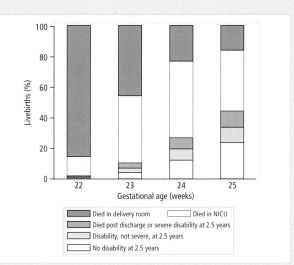

Fig. 2.3a Population-based study of mortality and disability in the UK and Ireland of all infants born alive at 22–25 weeks of gestation in 1995 at 30 months of age. EPICure Study. Wood NS *et al.* Neurologic and developmental disability after extremely preterm birth. *NEJM* 2000; **343**:378–384.

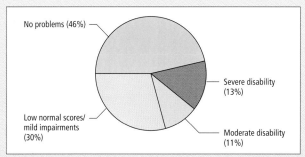

Fig. 2.3b Proportion of survivors of infants born alive at 22–25 weeks of gestation with disability at 6 years of age using standard definitions. (Adapted from Marlow N *et al.* for the EPICure Study Group. Neurologic and developmental disability at six years of age after extremely preterm birth. *NEJM* 2005; **352**: 9–19.)

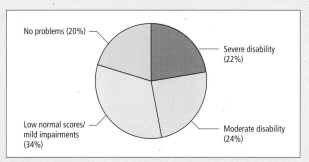

Fig. 2.3c Proportion of survivors with disability at 6 years of age defined by comparison with other children in their class. (Adapted from Marlow N *et al.* for the EPICure Study Group. Neurologic and developmental disability at six years of age after extremely preterm birth. *NEJM* 2005; **352**: 9–19.)

Epidemiologic data collection

Neonatal epidemiologic data are gathered from neonatal databases such as the Vermont–Oxford Neonatal network and NICHD (National Institute of Child Health and Human Development) Neonatal Research Network, which collect clinical data from a large number of neonatal units. Particularly informative are the population-based databases (Fig. 2.3a, b, c), some of which combine obstetric and neonatal data with outcome data (Fig. 2.4).

Infant mortality

The marked reduction in infant mortality since 1980 is shown in Fig. 2.2. With the decline in deaths from infectious diseases since the 1900s and more recently from sudden infant death syndrome, infant mortality is now mainly related to perinatal conditions (Fig. 2.5). Sixty-six per cent of all infant deaths occur in the 7.6% of infants born with low birthweight; 52% of infant deaths are among the 1.4% very low birthweight infants.

Compared with other countries, the US had only the 26th lowest infant mortality rate in 2000 (UK had the 21st lowest). A major reason for this relatively poor performance is the higher percentage of low birthweight infants born in the US than many other developed countries. It is also influenced by ethnicity: the mortality of infants of black mothers is 2.5 times higher than that of infants of white or Hispanic mothers.

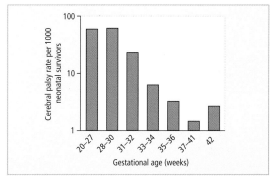

Fig. 2.4 Cerebral palsy by gestational age (Western Australia, 1980–1992), an example of population-based data combining perinatal data with outcome. (Source: Stanley F, Blair E, Alberman E. *Cerebral Palsies: Epidemiology and Causal Pathways*. London: Mac Keith Press, 2000.)

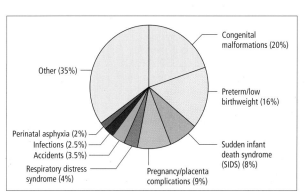

Fig. 2.5 Causes of infant mortality in the US, 2001. (Source: United States National Center for Health Statistics.)

The concept of perinatal care has evolved recently from the development of maternal–fetal medicine (fetal medicine and high-risk obstetrics) linked to neonatal intensive care and associated pediatric specialities. As the expertise required is highly specialized, rapidly advancing and multidisciplinary, it is usually provided centrally as a tertiary service, though some services may be available locally (Fig. 3.1).

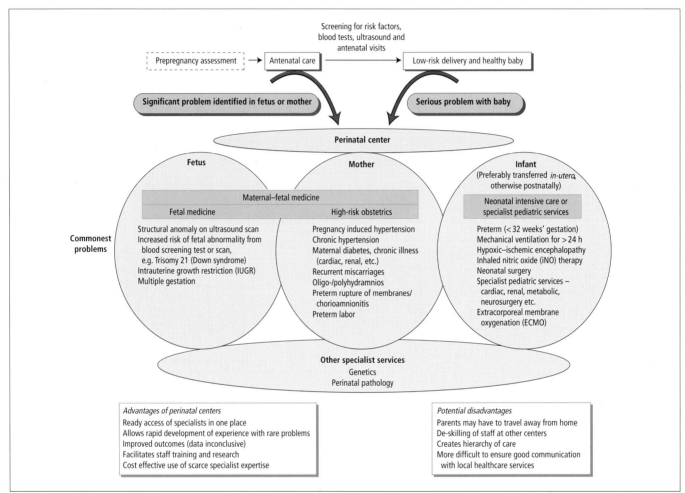

Fig 3.1 Organization of tertiary perinatal care.

Neonatal involvement in perinatal care

An increasing number of neonatal conditions requiring neonatal intensive care or specialist pediatric services are recognized antenatally. This allows transfer, if necessary, before birth to a perinatal center (Fig. 3.2). Parents require information about their baby's condition and management options. Neonatologists, specialist pediatricians and pediatric surgeons are now often involved to provide information before the baby is born. However, interpretation of ultrasound scans may be difficult antenatally, adding to the problem of providing parents with accurate information about the likely prognosis. Specialist assessment and counseling needs to be particularly prompt if termination of pregnancy is considered.

Information about problems identified antenatally needs to be communicated to the neonatologist or pediatrician so that appropriate assessment and follow-up are arranged after birth.

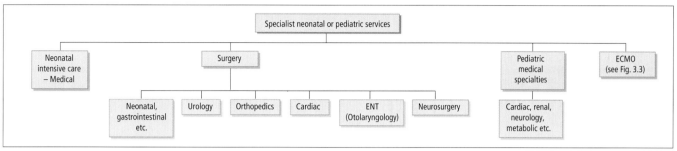

Fig. 3.2 Specialist neonatal care.

Levels of neonatal care

The different levels of care required by newborn infants are shown in Fig. 3.4.

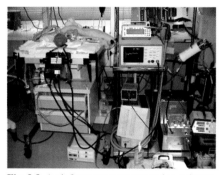

Fig. 3.3 An infant on extracorporeal membrane oxygenation (ECMO), which is provided at only a relatively small number of specialist centers.

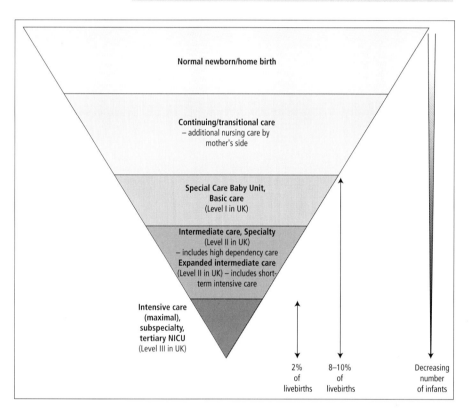

Fig. 3.4 Levels of neonatal care.

Prepregnancy care

Aim is to identify pregnancies at increased risk of fetal abnormality:
- mother >35 years old for trisomy 21 (Down syndrome)
- previous abnormal child
- family history of an inherited disorder
- consanguinous relationship
- parents known carriers of an autosomal recessive disorder, e.g. thalassemia
- parents from ethnic group with specific risk, e.g. Black-African American (sickle cell disease); Ashkenazi Jews (Tay–Sachs disease, a neurodegenerative disorder)
- a parent with known chromosomal rearrangement. Identification allows genetic counseling and advice about antenatal diagnosis.

Aim is to provide advice to optimize chances of healthy baby:
- attend clinic for prenatal care.
- avoid maternal smoking, alcohol, drug misuse, medication (unless essential).
- Toxoplasmosis exposure – avoid eating undercooked meat (and wear gloves when handling cat litter).
- *Listeria* infection – avoid unpasteurized dairy products and soft ripened cheeses, e.g. brie.
- take folic acid supplements to reduce risk of neural tube defects.
- check management of pre-existing maternal medical conditions, especially diabetes mellitus.

Prenatal screening

Maternal blood

The routine screening tests vary geographically, but include:
- blood group and antibodies for rhesus and other red cell incompatibilities
- hepatitis B and C
- syphilis
- rubella
- HIV infection
- neural tube defects – by maternal serum alphafetoprotein (MSAFP)
- trisomy 21 (Down syndrome) – a risk estimate is calculated by measuring three or more fetoplacental and maternal hormones and allowing for maternal age
- hemoglobin electrophoresis if indicated.

Cervical smear

Chlamydia (not done routinely in UK).

Ultrasound

Gestational age – reliable if at <20 weeks.

Multiple gestation – identified and chorionicity determined.

Structural malformations – can detect 30–70% of major congenital malformations.

Nuchal fold thickness in trisomy 21 (Down syndrome).

Fetal growth – monitored by serial measurement of abdominal circumference, head circumference and femur length.

Amniotic fluid volume
(i) oligohydramnios
  - from reduced fetal urine production, placental insufficiency and from prolonged rupture of the membranes
  - may cause pulmonary hypoplasia and limb and facial deformities from pressure on the fetus
(ii) polyhydramnios – associated with maternal diabetes, fetal bowel obstruction, CNS anomalies and multiple births.

Doppler studies – maternal and fetal circulation (if indicated).

Examples of structural malformations identified on ultrasound (Figs 4.1–3)

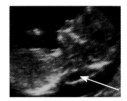

Fig. 4.1 Nuchal translucency (thickened fat pad at back of neck) associated with trisomy 21 (Down syndrome). (Courtesy of Ms Lorin Lakasing.)

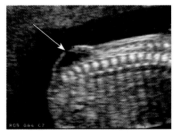

Fig. 4.2 Sacral myelocele. (Courtesy of Dr Venkhat Rahman.)

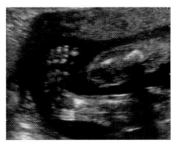

Fig. 4.3 Talipes equinovarus. (Courtesy of Dr Venkhat Rahman.)

Fetal medicine

Fetal medicine (Fig. 4.4) may allow:
• identification of congenital disorders
• option of termination of pregnancy to be offered for severe disorders

• therapy to be given for a limited but increasing number of conditions, e.g. fetal arrythmias, intrauterine blood transfusion for rhesus disease
• optimal obstetric management of the fetus, e.g. timing of delivery
• neonatal management to be planned in advance, e.g. counseling and transfer to specialty center.

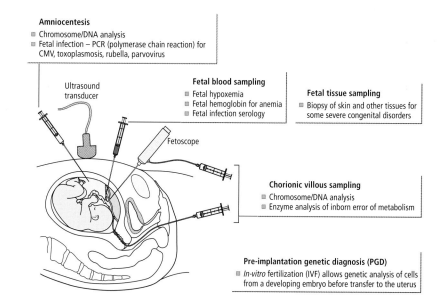

Amniocentesis
▪ Chromosome/DNA analysis
▪ Fetal infection – PCR (polymerase chain reaction) for CMV, toxoplasmosis, rubella, parvovirus

Ultrasound transducer

Fetal blood sampling
▪ Fetal hypoxemia
▪ Fetal hemoglobin for anemia
▪ Fetal infection serology

Fetal tissue sampling
▪ Biopsy of skin and other tissues for some severe congenital disorders

Fetoscope

Chorionic villous sampling
▪ Chromosome/DNA analysis
▪ Enzyme analysis of inborn error of metabolism

Pre-implantation genetic diagnosis (PGD)
▪ *In-vitro* fertilization (IVF) allows genetic analysis of cells from a developing embryo before transfer to the uterus

Fig. 4.4 Techniques in fetal medicine and their indications.

Fetal surgery

Creates media headlines as cutting-edge technology. However, the results are mostly poor as the malformations justifying fetal surgery are so severe and the risk of premature onset of labor is high. Now practiced only in a few centers and mainly restricted to randomized trials. With uterine surgery at early gestation there are concerns about adverse effect on future pregnancies. Cases must be carefully selected and detailed follow-up results collected and published.

Surgery
Performed at hysterotomy (uterus opened at 22–24 weeks' gestation) for diaphragmatic hernia and spina bifida. May precipitate preterm delivery, outcome disappointing.

In Europe, a trial of fetal treatment of diaphragmatic hernia is under way. As tracheal obstruction promotes lung growth, this is produced in the fetus by inflating a balloon in the trachea, inserted by tracheal intubation at fetoscopy.

Relief of urinary outflow obstruction
Catheter from bladder to amniotic cavity. Disappointing results.

Catheter shunts
Inserted under ultrasound guidance, for fetal pleural effusions, usually a chylothorax (lymphatic fluid) (Fig. 4.5). One end of a looped catheter lies in the chest, the other end in the amniotic cavity. Neonatal course often satisfactory.

Dilatation of stenotic heart valves
Via a transabdominal catheter inserted under ultrasound guidance into the fetal heart.

Shunting of hydrocephalus
Abandoned because of increased rate of severe disability.

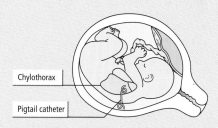

Chylothorax

Pigtail catheter

Fig. 4.5 Fetus with pigtail catheter to drain a pleural effusion.

Diabetes mellitus

Fetal mortality and morbidity are increased with maternal insulin-dependent diabetes (type 1), mainly from congenital malformations and intrauterine death. Good diabetic control, from preconception onwards, reduces malformations and mortality. This requires multidisciplinary management and close prenatal surveillance. The aim is for delivery at 38–40 weeks, by induction if necessary.

Fetal problems

• Congenital malformations. Risk 6%, four times normal. Wide spectrum of malformations but specific increased risk of cardiac malformations and caudal regression syndrome (sacral agenesis).
• Macrosomia (Fig. 5.1). Maternal hyperglycemia results in fetal hyperinsulinemia, which promotes growth. 25% of infants of diabetic mothers are macrosomic, with a birth weight >4 kg, compared with 8% of infants of non-diabetic mothers.
• Macrosomia predisposes to cephalopelvic disproportion and increased risk of delivery-related complications, including birth injuries.
• Intrauterine growth restriction (IUGR). Threefold increase. Usually associated with maternal vascular disease.
• Polyhydramnios.
• Preterm labor. Occurs in 10%, either natural or induced.
• Intrauterine death – sudden, in third trimester. Less common with good diabetic control.

Neonatal problems

• Check for malformations and birth injuries.
• Hypoglycemia – common in first 48 hours due to hyperinsulinism. Monitor blood glucose before feeds until >45 mg% (>2.6 mmol/l).

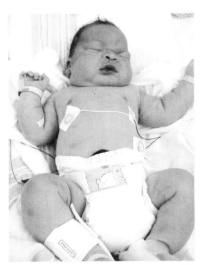

Fig. 5.1 Macrosomic infant with birth weight 4.8 kg at 38 weeks' gestation. There is excess fat and organomegaly (liver and heart).

Hypoglycemia is prevented by early, frequent feeding, but may require gavage (nasogastric) feeds or intravenous glucose. Hypocalcemia and hypomagnesemia are often present.
• Polycythemia – plethoric appearance. Occasionally requires partial exchange transfusion.
• Hyperbilirubinemia.
• Respiratory distress syndrome – increased risk from delayed maturation of surfactant.
• Hypertrophic cardiomyopathy – uncommon. Asymptomatic or poor cardiac output (may be treated with β-blockers) for several weeks.
• Renal vein thrombosis – rare.

Gestational diabetes

Glucose intolerance complicates 1–2% of pregnancies and may require dietary or insulin treatment. May cause neonatal macrosomia, hypoglycemia and polycythemia.

Red blood cell isoimmunization

Maternal antibody is formed to fetal red blood cell antigens, e.g. rhesus D, anti-Kell and anti-c. Before prophylaxis, rhesus disease was a major cause of fetal and neonatal morbidity and mortality.

Rhesus hemolytic disease

Etiology
See Fig. 5.2.

Presentation
• Antibodies found on routine antenatal antibody screen at first visit, 28 and 34 weeks.
• Previous pregnancy affected with hemolytic disease.
• Fetal hydrops on ultrasound
• Maternal polyhydramnios
• Infant – jaundice, anemia, hydrops, hepatosplenomegaly.

Management
PRENATAL
• Increasing antibody titres on screening – refer to specialist center if necessary.
• Monitor with serial ultrasound for fetal anemia and hydrops.
  If indicated:
• Amniocentesis – for amniotic fluid optical density (450 nm) to assess degree of hemolysis (now rarely used).
• Measure fetal hematocrit (from cord).
• Intrauterine blood transfusion.
• Deliver preterm if necessary.

POSTNATAL
• Check cord blood for blood type, hemoglobin, bilirubin and direct antibody test (DAT).

Etiology

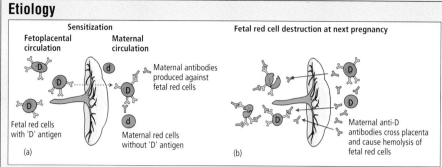

Fig. 5.2 (a) A small number of fetal red cells enter the maternal circulation and antibodies are formed. This usually occurs at delivery, but also at miscarriages, placental abruption, from blood transfusions and occasionally during normal pregnancies. (b) Maternal antibodies on re-exposure to fetal red cells at subsequent pregnancy cross the placenta and bind to fetal cells, causing hemolysis (see Table 5.1).

Table 5.1 Effect of hemolysis.

Fetus
Anemia – progressive
Hepatosplenomegaly
Hydrops (edema, ascites)
Death
Infant
Anemia
Hyperbilirubinemia

- Monitor bilirubin closely as level may increase rapidly and cause high-frequency deafness or kernicterus.
- Start intensive phototherapy and do exchange transfusion if severe anemia or rapidly rising bilirubin.
- May need blood transfusion for anemia at several weeks of age.

Prevention
Anti-D gammaglobulin has almost eliminated rhesus disease. It is given to rhesus-negative mothers during pregnancy, after potentially sensitizing events, and after delivery.

15% of Caucasian women are rhesus-negative; less than 2% of them become sensitized because of inadequate or failed prophylaxis.

Perinatal isoimmune thrombocytopenia

Analogous to rhesus disease – maternal antibodies (HPLA1 in 80%) directed against fetal platelets cross the placenta. Affects 1 in 5000 births. Intracranial hemorrhage secondary to fetal thrombocytopenia occurs in up to 25%, occasionally antenatally. If identified from a previously affected infant, prevention is by repeated intrauterine platelet transfusions.

Thrombocytopenia after birth is treated with platelets that are negative for the platelet antigen. The role of intravenous immunoglobulin (IVIG) is uncertain. The thrombocytopenia may persist for several weeks.

Other maternal medical conditions (Table 5.2)

Table 5.2 Other maternal medical conditions that may affect the infant.

Maternal condition	Significance for the infant
Maternal hyperthyroidism	If mother is controlled on treatment, fetus and infant are usually unaffected. Rarely causes:
	Transient hyperthyroidism – fetal tachycardia, and neonatal hyperthyroidism (1–3%) – tachycardia, heart failure, vomiting, diarrhea and failure to thrive (despite good intake), jitteriness, goiter and exophthalmos (protuberant eyes). Treated for 2–3 months
	Transient hypothyroidism – from maternal drug therapy
Maternal hypothyroidism	Worldwide; commonest cause is iodine deficiency. Important cause of congenital hypothyroidism, leading to short stature and severe learning difficulties. Rarely seen in the US or UK
	Mothers treated with thyroxine; neonatal problems are rare
Autoimmune thrombocytopenic purpura (AITP)	Maternal autoantibodies against platelet surface antigens cross the placenta and cause fetal thrombocytopenia. Can be treated *in utero* with repeated intravenous platelet transfusions. If severe, may cause cerebral hemorrhage before birth or from birth trauma, but this is rare. Infants with severe thrombocytopenia or petechiae at birth should be given intravenous immunoglobulin. Platelet transfusions are reserved for platelet count <20 000 mm³ (20×10^9/L) or active bleeding because of the anti-platelet antibodies. The platelet count declines over the first few days before increasing
Systemic lupus erythematosus (SLE)	Intrauterine growth restriction, preterm delivery; rarely causes a lupus rash and complete heart block in the fetus (from antibodies to the Ro and La antigen)

Importance

The prenatal identification of the intrauterine growth restriction (IUGR) is important because it allows:
- timely delivery of the fetus with chronic hypoxia, who is at risk of intrauterine death
- early identification of serious fetal abnormalities and fetal infection.

The neonate is at risk of:
- birth asphyxia
- hypoglycemia because of poor reserves of glycogen and other energy sources, e.g. fat
- polycythemia from intrauterine hypoxia
- hypothermia
- mortality.

During childhood most show catch-up growth, but some remain short and thin. There is a slight increase in risk of learning difficulties with IUGR.

Definition

IUGR is the failure of a fetus or infant to achieve his or her genetic growth potential. Most will also be small for gestational age (SGA), although the two terms are not synonymous. SGA means that the infant is below a particular weight centile for gestation; the 10th centile is most often chosen, but the 3rd or other centiles are also used (Fig. 6.1). The higher the centile chosen, the higher the proportion of infants included who are normal but small; the lower the centile used the higher the proportion with a pathologic cause, but more will be missed. The fetus may have growth failure but may not be SGA as their weight is still above the 10th centile.

Etiology

Fetal

- Chromosomal disorders, e.g. trisomy 18 and other genetic syndromes.
- Structural malformations.
- Congenital infection – CMV, toxoplasmosis, rubella.

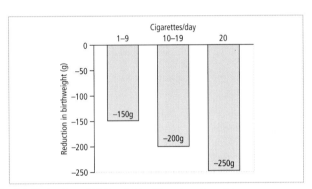

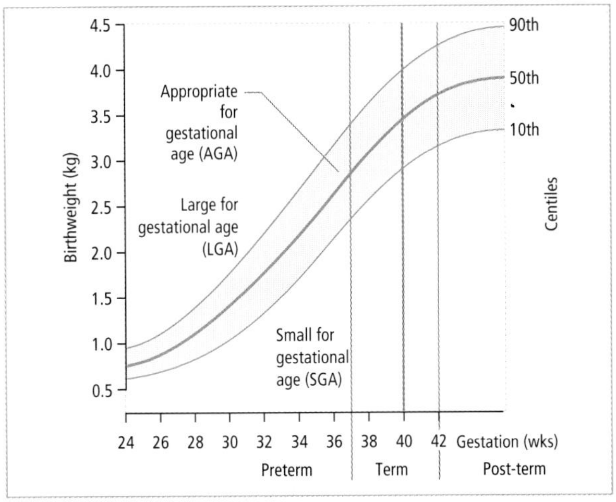

Fig. 6.2 Reduction of birthweight with maternal smoking.

Maternal

- Undernutrition, e.g. famine in developing countries, eating disorders.
- Maternal hypoxia, e.g. cyanotic heart disease, chronic respiratory disease, altitude.
- Drugs, e.g. cigarettes (Fig. 6.2), alcohol, illicit.

Placental

- Reduced maternal vascular supply – pre-eclampsia, chronic maternal disease, e.g. hypertension, diabetes mellitus, renal disease.
- Thrombosis, infarction, e.g. maternal lupus anticoagulant, antiphospholipid syndrome, sickle cell disease.
- Sharing of uterine vascularity – multiple gestation.

Pathophysiology

Traditionally, IUGR has been classified as symmetric or asymmetric, though in clinical practice there is considerable overlap.
- **Symmetric** – growth failure affecting weight, head and length. Caused by fetal factors, e.g. chromosomal disorders, syndromes or congenital infection. May be accompanied by polyhydramnios if there is reduced fetal swallowing of amniotic fluid, e.g. trisomy 21 (Down syndrome), gastrointestinal obstruction. The infant is likely to continue to be small throughout childhood.

Fig. 6.1 Chart showing increase in birthweight with gestational age. Most small for gestational age fetuses or infants are constitutionally small.

- **Asymmetric** – growth failure with head (reflecting brain) growth relatively preserved. Caused by uteroplacental insufficiency with reduced oxygen transfer to the fetus. Fetal adaptation to hypoxia is to preserve blood supply to the vital organs, i.e. the brain, myocardium and adrenal glands, at the expense of the kidney, gastrointestinal tract and liver, limbs and subcutaneous tissues. This is reflected in maintained head growth but reduced abdominal circumference from reduced glycogen stores in the liver and oligohydramnios from reduced urine production. If it progresses, it results in fetal acidemia and fetal death.

Management

Management is intensive fetal surveillance to maximize gestation without compromising the fetus (Fig. 6.3).

Antenatal

- Establish if there is a fetal cause by detailed ultrasound scanning for fetal anomalies and karyotype if indicated.
- Monitor fetal growth and well-being from measurements of growth parameters, biophysical profile (amniotic fluid volume, fetal movement, fetal tone, fetal breathing movements, fetal heart activity) and Doppler blood flow velocity. Deliver, depending on gestational age, if growth ceases or abnormal biophysical profile or significant abnormality of the Doppler flow velocity waveform (Fig. 6.4).

Postnatal

- After birth, the infant is monitored for hypoglycemia and polycythemia and examined for evidence of dysmorphic features or congenital infection.

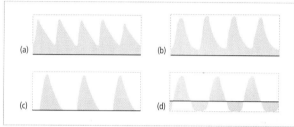

Fig. 6.4 Umbilical Doppler waveform. Normal (a), end diastolic flow velocity reduced (b), absent (c), reversed (d). Doppler signals from the umbilical artery give information about fetoplacental blood flow. Increased blood flow velocities in the fetal middle cerebral artery and absent or reversed flow in diastole in the fetal aorta indicates fetal hypoxia. Reversed end-diastolic flow in the ductus venosus indicates fetal myocardial insufficiency and the need for delivery.

Question

What is the significance of birth weight in adult life?

There is considerable evidence that infants of low birthweight are at higher risk of NIDDM (non-insulin-dependent diabetes mellitus, type 2), coronary heart disease, hypertension and stroke (Barker hypothesis). However, postnatal environmental factors are more important.

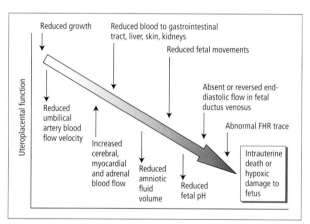

Fig. 6.3 Consequences of progressive uteroplacental failure.

Preterm delivery

About 7–12% of deliveries in developed countries are preterm (12% in US, 7% in UK). The proportion of infants born preterm has increased as a result of assisted reproductive technology and medical intervention for fetal or medical reasons.

The causes of preterm delivery are shown in Fig. 7.1. The aim is to prolong pregnancy for as long as possible while ensuring the safety of the mother and fetus. The decision to deliver preterm is most difficult at the limit of viability, at 23–26 weeks of gestation, and should involve the obstetrician, neonatologist and parents. Decision-making is helped by a detailed assessment of fetal well-being, including assessment of liquor volume, fetal heart rate monitoring and Doppler studies, fetal growth, gestation and predicted birth weight (with estimates of their accuracy). Decision-making will also be informed by knowledge of the morbidity and mortality at these early gestational ages. National data are available, but will need to be modified according to the outcomes for each individual neonatal unit.

Key points

- Corticosteroids should be given to mothers at 24–34 weeks of gestation if at high risk of preterm labor to promote fetal lung maturation.
- Tocolytics are sometimes given to the mother to attempt to delay delivery to allow the corticosteroids to work or to facilitate *in utero* transfer to a perinatal center.
- Delivery of high-risk infants should preferably occur at a specialty center to avoid subsequent transfer and separation of the infant and mother.
- Neonatal care of preterm infants is very expensive. The typical cost of intensive care is $2400 (£1300) per day, basic (special) care $1500 (£800) per day. Preterm infants are likely to be in hospital until about 2 weeks before their expected date of delivery, but sometimes considerably longer.
- 26% of infants of birthweight <1500 g are multiple births (NICHD Neonatal Research Network, 2002).

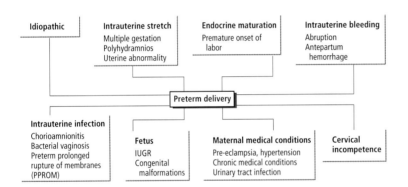

Fig. 7.1 Causes of prematurity. IUGR, intrauterine growth restriction; PPROM, preterm prolonged rupture of the membranes.

Multiple births

The incidence of spontaneous multiple gestation in Caucasian populations is:
- 1 in 89 for twins
- 1 in 89^2 (1 in 8000) for triplets
- 1 in 89^3 (1 in 700 000) for quadruplets.

However, the number of multiple gestations has increased because of the older age of childbearing and assisted reproduction pregnancies, 20% of which are multiple (Fig. 7.2). As a result, 1 in 69 births is now a multiple birth. The high number of triplets and higher-order births has declined in the UK as the maximum number of embryos transferred has been restricted to three, with two recommended. In the US there are recommendations that triplet and higher-order multiple births are avoided and their number has plateaued.

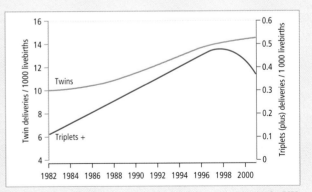

Fig. 7.2 Increase in number of multiple-gestation deliveries in the UK.

Pregnancy complications

Twins may:
- have their own chorionic sac and placenta (dichorionic, 67%)
- share a chorionic sac and placenta (monochorionic, 33%).

The main pregnancy complications of twins are:

- **Preterm delivery.** The increased prematurity rate (Fig. 7.3) is responsible for the increase in perinatal mortality, which for twins is six times that of singletons.
- **Intrauterine growth restriction (IUGR).** Affects 20% of dichorionic twins and 40% of monochorionic twins. If one twin has IUGR, the potential benefits of early delivery of that twin have to be weighed against the prematurity-related complications of the normally grown twin. Intrauterine death of a twin may result in neurologic impairment or death of the surviving twin if monochorionic.
- **Congenital abnormalities.** In dichorionic twins the risk is 2 times normal, as there are two infants. However, in monochorionic twins the risk is 4 times normal.
- **Twin–twin transfusion syndrome (TTTS).** This occurs in some monochorionic twin pregnancies across placental arteriovenous anastomoses. The donor develops anemia and hypovolemia from blood loss and growth restriction, and oliguria and oligohydramnios from placental insufficiency. The other twin experiences hypervolemia and polycythemia, which may result in high-output cardiac failure, polyuria and polyhydramnios. This may result in preterm labor or intrauterine death. Potential *in utero* treatment includes laser therapy to coagulate the placental blood vessels or, rarely, periodic drainage of the amniotic fluid.
- **Death of a fetus.** Intrauterine death of a twin may result in preterm labor. In monochorionic twins, there may be blood loss from the live to the dead twin, leading to hypovolemia, neurologic impairment or death of the surviving twin.

Neonatal complications

For multiple preterm births, the immediate problem is to find sufficient intensive care beds and staff. Every effort should be made to avoid sending the infants to different units.

Apart from prematurity, other immediate medical problems may be from twin–twin transfusion syndrome (anemia may require blood or exchange transfusion; polycythemia may require exchange transfusion), intrauterine growth restriction and congenital malformations. It is more difficult, but often possible, to fully breast-feed twins but not higher-order births.

Families of multiple births may need additional assistance and support:

- practical – with their care and housework (requires about 200 hours/week for triplets in infancy!), may require help to be able to leave the house (Fig. 7.4)
- emotional – exhausting to provide care
- privacy – loss of privacy as a couple
- financial – considerable additional costs (cannot hand down clothes or equipment), may need rehousing
- increased incidence of parental depression, especially if there was fetal or neonatal loss (when every birthday or other achievement of the survivor is a reminder that the co-twin died)
- behavioral – problems in other siblings is increased threefold
- development – reduced opportunities for mother–infant interaction, as mothers are busy and often tired. Increased risk of delayed language development and poor attention span. While multiple births may provide companionship, affection and stimulation between each other, they may also engender domination, dependency and jealousy.

There are local and national support groups for parents of multiple births.

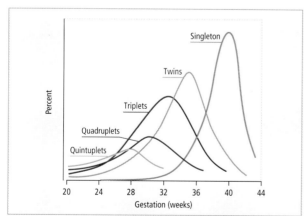

Fig. 7.3 Schematic diagram to show gestational age distribution at delivery of multiple births.

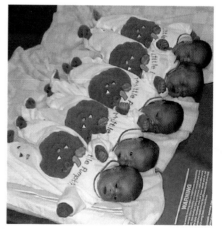

Fig. 7.4 Quintuplets. Multiple births look endearing but families may need assistance with their care.

8 Birth defects and genetic disorders

The causes of birth defects are shown in Table 8.1. The mechanisms by which they arise are shown in Fig. 8.1. When confronted with an infant with a birth defect, there are a number of questions one needs to ask (Table 8.2), features one needs to look for (Table 8.3) and investigations to consider (Table 8.4).

Table 8.1 Causes of birth defects.

Teratogenic	Environmental agents during pregnancy – infections, drugs (particularly anticonvulsants), alcohol and radiation
Sporadic or multifactorial	Many single birth defects occur as isolated cases with low recurrence risk. These may be polygenic or due to faults in developmental pathways
Single-gene disorders	May be family history and previous pregnancy losses. Many multiple malformation syndromes follow autosomal recessive inheritance, but consider X-linked recessive disorders in males and new dominant mutations in isolated cases
Chromosomal	Usually cause multiple congenital malformations and learning difficulties

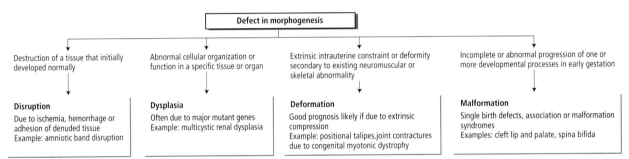

Fig. 8.1 Mechanisms of birth defects.

Table 8.2 What to ask about.

Parental age and health
Previous reproductive history
Family history of birth defects
Consanguinity
Exposure to potential teratogens
Complications during pregnancy
Ultrasound screening and further investigations
Fetal movements

Table 8.3 What to look for.

Growth parameters	Intrauterine growth restriction, overgrowth, microcephaly
Movement and posture	Hypotonia, contractures, seizures
Minor anomalies	Features with little cosmetic or functional significance. The presence of 2 or more should prompt a search for major anomalies
Major birth defects	May represent an association (defects occurring together more often than by chance alone). e.g. VACTERL (vertebral, anal atresia, cardiac, tracheo-esophageal fistula, renal and limb) May represent a sequence (one initial malformation resulting in the development of others, e.g. renal agenesis resulting in Potter sequence) May represent a syndrome (defects occurring together which have a common, specific etiology)
Dysmorphic features	Unusual or distinctive external appearance of the face, hands, feet, etc.

Table 8.4 Investigations to consider.

Clinical photographs	Provide a valuable record, especially if the phenotype changes with time
Chromosome analysis	Order chromosome analysis (karyotype) in all babies with multiple malformations or dysmorphic features. Consider requesting FISH (fluorescence in situ hybridization) tests for specific disorders, such as Williams syndrome, if appropriate
Biochemical analysis	Examples are calcium (for suspected Williams syndrome or DiGeorge syndrome) and creatinine kinase (for suspected congenital muscular dystrophy)
Skeletal survey	Suspected skeletal dysplasia, such as achondroplasia
Echocardiography	Suspected congenital heart disease
Renal ultrasound	If renal anomalies suspected, e.g. in some chromosomal disorders
Brain CT/MRI/ultrasound scan	Suspected CNS malformation
Molecular analysis	Specific disorders, e.g. cystic fibrosis, spinal muscular atrophy type 1

Chromosomal disorders

Trisomy 21 (Down syndrome)

Incidence is 1 in 650 live births. Most cases (94%) are due to non-disjunction of chromosome 21 during meiosis in the formation of eggs or sperm (Fig. 8.2). The risk increases with maternal age (Table 8.5).

About 5% of cases are due to translocation, in which chromosome 21 is translocated onto another chromosome (usually onto chromosome 14). The risk of trisomy 21 is about 10% when the balanced translocation is carried by the mother.

Clinical features

Trisomy 21 is not always identified on prenatal screening with ultrasound or maternal blood testing. The facial appearance (Fig. 8.3a) and other clinical signs (Fig 8.3b–c) are usually recognizable at birth but diagnosis needs to be confirmed by chromosome analysis. Associated malformations include congenital heart disease, duodenal atresia and Hirschsprung disease.

Subsequently there is increased risk of:

- learning difficulties
- small stature
- secretory otitis media and hearing impairment
- visual impairment
- leukemia
- hypothyroidism
- Alzheimer disease.

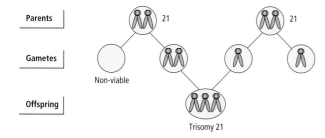

Fig. 8.2 Trisomy 21 due to non-disjunction.

Table 8.5 Risk of trisomy 21 in liveborn infants by maternal age.

Maternal age at delivery (years)	Risk
All ages	1 in 650
30	1 in 900
35	1 in 400
37	1 in 250
39	1 in 150
40	1 in 100
44	1 in 40

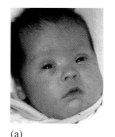
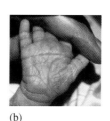
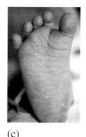

(a)   (b)   (c)

Fig. 8.3 Trisomy 21 (Down syndrome). (a) Facial features – upward slant of eyes, epicanthic folds, low set simple ears, flat occiput, third fontanelle, short neck. (b) Hands – single palmar crease and short little finger. (c) Feet – wide gap between first and second toes. Other features – hypotonia.

Trisomy 18 (Edwards syndrome)

Incidence is 0.1/1000 live births.

Most infants have intrauterine growth restriction (birth weight 1.5–2.5 kg at term). Dysmorphic features include prominent occiput, narrow forehead, small mouth and jaw, short sternum, clenched hands with overlapping digits (Fig. 8.4a), prominent heels and rocker-bottom feet (Fig. 8.4b). Major malformations include heart defects, neural tube defects, omphalocele, esophageal atresia and radial defects. Most die shortly after birth.

Trisomy 13 (Patau syndrome)

Incidence is around 0.7/1000 live births.

Dysmorphic features include scalp defects (Fig. 8.5a), broad nasal tip and polydactyly. Major malformations include holoprosencephaly (brain is a single hemisphere), microcephaly, ocular malformations, cleft lip and palate (Fig. 8.5b), heart defects and renal abnormality. Most babies die within 1 month.

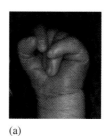
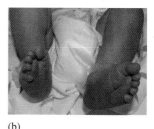

(a)   (b)

Fig. 8.4 Characteristic abnormalities of trisomy 18 (Edwards syndrome). (a) Typical clenched hand with overlying digits. (b) Rocker-bottom feet.

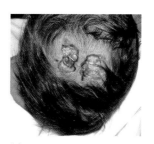
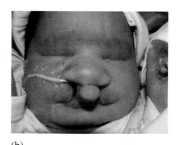

(a)   (b)

Fig. 8.5 Characteristic abnormalities of trisomy 13 (Patau syndrome). (a) Scalp defect. (b) Cleft lip and palate.

Almost all fetuses are exposed to one or more of the following potential toxins:
- over-the-counter medications
- prescription drugs
- diagnostic agents (e.g. X-rays)
- recreational drugs, e.g. cigarettes, alcohol or illicit drugs
- herbal and vitamin supplements
- environmental exposure (e.g. pollutants).

The potential consequences for the fetus are listed in Table 9.1.

Table 9.1 Potential consequences for the fetus of perinatal drug exposure.

Intrauterine growth restriction
Intrauterine death or abortion
Recognizable patterns of congenital anomalies
Maladaptation to extrauterine life
Neonatal withdrawal syndrome
Toxic effects due to passage of drugs into breast milk
Delayed effects on neurodevelopment and behavior

Maternal smoking

In the fetus, maternal cigarette smoking is associated with:
- increased risk of miscarriage and stillbirth
- reduction in birthweight, with increase in intrauterine growth restriction (IUGR) related to number cigarettes smoked per day, with average birth weight reduction of 170 g at term.

In the infant it is associated with:
- increased risk of sudden infant death syndrome (SIDS)
- increased wheezing in childhood.

Alcohol

Severe prolonged maternal alcohol ingestion is associated with fetal alcohol syndrome (FAS) (Fig 9.1). The American Academy of Pediatrics recommends abstinence. The effect of occasional, mild alcohol ingestion or occasional binge drinking is not known.

Figure 9.1 shows features of fetal alcohol syndrome.

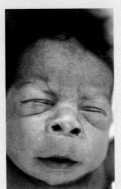

Features of fetal alcohol syndrome:
- Characteristic facies
  - saddle-shaped nose
  - maxillary hypoplasia
  - absent philtrum (ridges between the nose and upper lip)
  - thin upper lip
- Symmetric growth failure – severe, persistent
- Cardiac defects (40–50%)
- Behavior problems – irritable in infancy, hyperactive in childhood
- Developmental delay – average I.Q. 63

Fig. 9.1 Features of fetal alcohol syndrome. (Photograph courtesy of Dr David Clark.)

Neonatal withdrawal (abstinence) syndrome

- Serious problem because of widespread use of narcotics and other drugs of dependency.
- Situation often complicated by multiple drug use.
- Mothers on heroin are usually encouraged to change to methadone.
- Increased risk of hepatitis B and C and HIV infection if intravenous drug user.
- Onset of withdrawal:
  - heroin <2 days
  - methadone <2 days but can be delayed up to 2 weeks.
- Cocaine does not cause problems from withdrawal but from direct transfer of the drug:
  - placental infarction leading to fetal death, IUGR or placental abruption and antepartum hemorrhage
  - cerebral infarction *in utero*.

Clinical assessment

This must be done systematically and repeatedly (6 hourly) (Table 9.2). This is facilitated by using a scoring system (e.g. Finnegan's score) to determine whether therapy is required. In some centers, analysis of meconium is performed to determine drug exposure during pregnancy.

Treatment

Usually with oral morphine sulfate, aiming to wean by titration of dose with score.

Medical and social services discharge planning meetings are often required during pregnancy and after birth as the lifestyle of many drug users is not conducive to the care of babies and children.

Table 9.2 Clinical features of opiate withdrawal.

Irritability	Vomiting
Scratching	Diarrhea
Wakefulness	Yawning
Shrill cry	Hiccoughs
Tremors	Salivation
Hypertonicity	Stuffy nose
Seizures	Sneezing
Pyrexia >38°C	Sweating
Tachypnea (rate >60/min)	Dehydration

Key point

Consider drug withdrawal (abstinence) if an infant has some of these clinical features and no cause has been identified.

Table 9.3 Some recognizable patterns of malformation or neonatal problems following maternal drug ingestion.

Time in pregnancy	Drug	Malformations/problems	Drug	Malformations/problems
Organogenesis (<8 weeks gestation)	**Thalidomide**	Short limbs (Fig. 9.2) Absent auricles, deafness	**Folic acid inhibitors** (methotrexate) as cytotoxic therapy	Fetal syndrome – microcephaly, neural tube defects, short limbs
	Anticonvulsants: • carbamazepine • valproic acid (sodium valproate) • hydantoins (phenytoin)	Fetal carbamazepine/ valproate/hydantoin syndrome – midfacial hypoplasia, CNS, limb and cardiac malformations Developmental delay	**Coumarin** (warfarin)	Fetal coumarin (warfarin) syndrome – nasal hypoplasia, microcephaly, hydrocephalus, optic atrophy, congenital heart defects, stippled epiphyses, purpuric rash
Pregnancy (>8 weeks' gestation)	**Antithyroid drugs** (iodides, propylthiouracil) **Androgens**	Goiter Congenital hypothyroidism Masculinization of female	**Tetracyclines** **β-blockers and hypoglycemic agents**	Hypoplasia of tooth enamel, yellow–brown staining of teeth Neonatal hypoglycemia
	Aspirin/non-steroidal anti-inflammatory drugs	Closure of ductus arteriosus in fetus		
Labor and delivery	Opiate analgesia	Respiratory depression at birth		

Medicines

Relatively few medicines produce recognizable patterns of malformation in the fetus (Table 9.3). Adverse effects may not be recognized if they are subtle or have delayed presentation, e.g. diethylstilbestrol (DES) given for threatened miscarriage in the mother and subsequent association with clear-cell adenocarcinoma of the vagina and cervix in female offspring, evident only during adolescence or early adult life.

Pregnant women should avoid taking both prescribed and over-the-counter medications whenever possible. For prescribed drugs, the benefits must outweigh the risks and appropriate maternal and fetal surveillance undertaken.

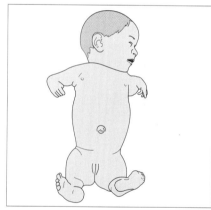

Fig. 9.2 Severe limb shortening (phocomelia, 'like a seal') from maternal thalidomide therapy, which was widely marketed (not in US) for morning sickness from 1957. Teratogenic effects only recognized several years later.

The term 'congenital infection' applies to infections acquired *in utero* (Fig. 10.1) whereas 'neonatal infection' is acquired shortly before or at delivery or postnatally (see Chapter 40).

Most congenital infections are viral, but other causes include toxoplasmosis and syphilis.

Maternal infection is usually primary, i.e. it is a first infection, when there is lack of maternal immunity. Infection from recurrent maternal infection (e.g. with CMV or HSV) is usually less severe than from a primary infection. Maternal infection may be asymptomatic.

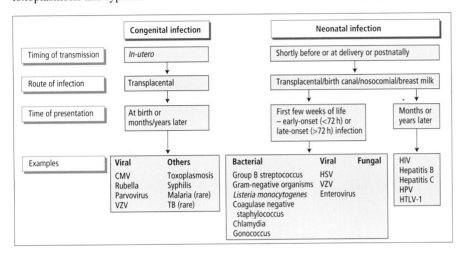

Fig. 10.1 Congenital and neonatal infections. (CMV – cytomegalovirus; VZV – varicella-zoster virus; HSV – herpes simplex virus; HPV – human papilloma virus; HTLV-1 – Human T cell leukemia virus 1.)

Clinical features

Congenital infections may precipitate abortion, stillbirth or pre-term delivery. The clinical features of the symptomatic infant are shown in Fig. 10.2.

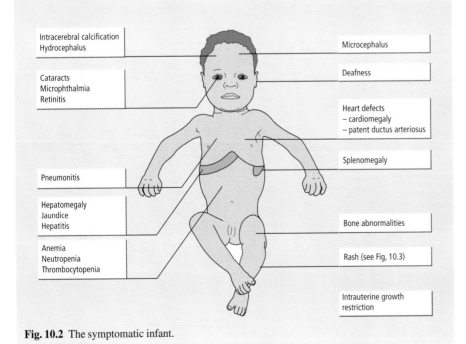

Fig. 10.2 The symptomatic infant.

Key point

It is not possible to reliably tell clinically if the cause is CMV, toxoplasmosis, rubella or syphilis.

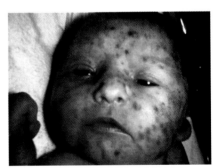

Fig. 10.3 Blueberry muffin rash.

Diagnosis (Table 10.1)

Table 10.1 Diagnosis of congenital infection.

Antenatal	Postnatal
	Maternal History (e.g. rash, contact) Screening serology – seroconversion (IgG, IgM, IgA) Culture/PCR of lesion, e.g. cervical herpes, blood, urine
Fetal Ultrasound scanning for anomalies Amniocentesis for fluid or fetal blood sample for serology/culture/PCR	**Placenta** Histology/microscopic dark-field examination for spirochetes in syphilis Culture/PCR
	Infant Culture/PCR – blood, urine, CSF, stool, nasopharyngeal aspirate, skin lesions Early serology may not help, as seroconversion may be delayed

PCR, polymerase chain reaction.

Congenital cytomegalovirus (CMV) infection

- Commonest congenital infection in the US and UK (0.5–1/1000 livebirths). Even more prevalent in developing countries.
- 1–2% of mothers seroconvert during pregnancy.
- Transmission is more likely the later the maternal seroconversion.
- Overall mother-to-infant transmission rate is 40%.
- May be transmitted in breast milk or blood transfusions.

Infected infants

- 5–10% severely affected (Fig. 10.2).
- 80–90% asymptomatic.
- Poor prognosis if abnormalities detectable on antenatal ultrasound – microcephaly, periventricular calcification (Fig. 10.4), CNS translucencies, hyperechoic abdominal mass, hepatic lesions.
- Most common infectious cause of sensorineural hearing loss.

Diagnosis

- Viral isolation from urine, saliva.
- Viral DNA (by PCR amplification) from amniotic fluid, urine, CSF.

Treatment

For severely affected newborn:
- Ganciclovir (intravenous) will improve acute organ disease (eye, liver, bone marrow, lungs), but controversial whether it has long-term benefit for CNS damage.

Key points

- Although clinicians sometimes refer to TORCH (toxoplasmosis, other, rubella, cytomegalovirus, herpes) screening, a range of different tests is required.
- Collect samples as soon as possible to optimize chances of diagnosis.

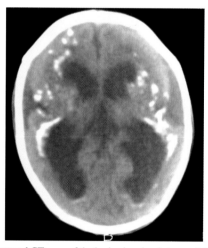

Fig. 10.4 Postnatal CT scan of the brain showing intracranial calcification from congenital CMV infection. The calcification may be identified on antenatal ultrasound.

Other points

- No vaccine yet for seronegative mothers.
- Infected infants have a persistently abnormal immune response to CMV.
- Infected infants may excrete CMV in urine for many months.

Congenital toxoplasmosis

- Usually after primary maternal infection in pregnancy.
- Seronegative mothers are most at risk from poorly cooked meat. Small risk from handling feces of recently infected cats or ingesting contaminated soil from unwashed vegetables.
- The transmission rate and treatment are shown in Table 10.2. The earlier in pregnancy the mother is infected the more severely the fetus is affected.
- The clinical features of the symptomatic infant are shown in Fig. 10.2. Subclinical disease includes retinitis (Fig. 10.5), epilepsy and learning difficulties.

Rubella

- Prevented by maternal vaccination. Now very rare in immunized populations.
- The earlier in pregnancy the mother is infected the more severely the fetus is affected.
- Clinical features are shown in Fig. 10.2.
- There is no effective treatment.

Table 10.2 Transmission rate and treatment of toxoplasmosis.

Trimester	Transmission rate	Clinical features	Treatment
First	15%	35% die before birth, 40% severely affected	Preventative – spiramycin
Second	40%		If severely affected – with antibiotics (pyrimethamine and sulfadiazine)
Third	60%	90% subclinical disease at birth; clinical manifestations may present years later	

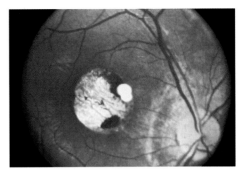

Fig. 10.5 Retinitis from toxoplasmosis. This may present many years later.

Congenital syphilis

In the US, a marked increase in incidence occurred in the 1980s, especially among drug users, but it has since declined. In the UK it is extremely rare. Antenatal screening on maternal blood is performed routinely. If active infection is diagnosed or suspected, the mother should be treated. Treatment more than 4 weeks before delivery prevents congenital infection.

- Transmission rate during primary infection in pregnancy is 100%.
- Without treatment there is 40% abortion/stillbirth/perinatal death.
- Clinical features are shown in Fig. 10.2. Those specific to congenital syphilis include a characteristic rash on the soles of the feet (Fig. 10.6) and hands (Fig. 10.7) and bone lesions (Fig. 10.8).

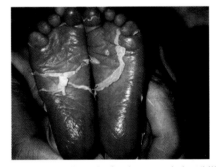

Fig. 10.6 Characteristic rash on the feet in congenital syphilis.

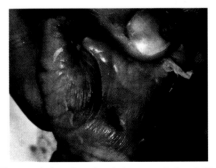

Fig. 10.7 Characteristic rash on hands in congenital syphilis.

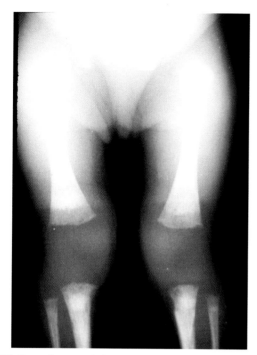

Fig. 10.8 X-rays in congenital syphilis showing bilateral metaphyseal lucency of the long bones and destruction of the medial proximal metaphysis of the left tibia.

- Treatment antenatally and/or postnatally is with penicillin. Effectiveness of treatment is monitored serologically.
- If the mother has not received adequate treatment or if there is physical, laboratory or radiographic evidence of disease, treat. If there is any doubt, treat directly.

Varicella: chickenpox, varicella zoster virus (VZV) infection

Primary maternal infection in pregnancy is uncommon as more than 90% of mothers are immune.

Early in pregnancy

- Intrauterine infection is rare (2% risk)
- Can lead to eye and CNS damage, skin scarring (Fig. 10.9) and limb hypoplasia.

Late in pregnancy

Infants born to mothers who develop chickenpox between 5 days before or 2 days after delivery should be given varicella zoster immune globulin (VZIG). This reduces but does not eliminate the risk of neonatal varicella zoster virus (VZV).

They should be closely monitored, and should be started on aciclovir (intravenous) if any signs of infection develop.

Parvovirus B19

- 50% of pregnant women are susceptible to infection.
- Transmission rate is 20–30%.
- In most cases there is a normal outcome of pregnancy but rarely:
  - infection in early pregnancy can lead to fetal loss
  - infection later in pregnancy can lead to severe fetal anemia (aplastic anemia), causing hydrops fetalis (edema and ascites from heart failure). May require an intrauterine exchange transfusion for the severe anemia.

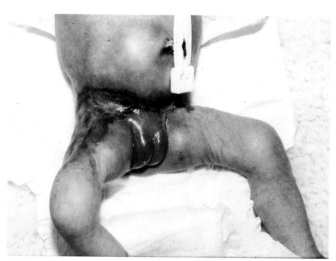

Fig. 10.9 Skin scarring from maternal VZV infection early in pregnancy. This is rare.

The transition from intrauterine to extrauterine life involves a complex sequence of physiologic changes that begin before birth. Remarkably, although infants experience some degree of intermittent hypoxemia during labor, most undergo this transition uneventfully. If not, prompt resuscitation will be required.

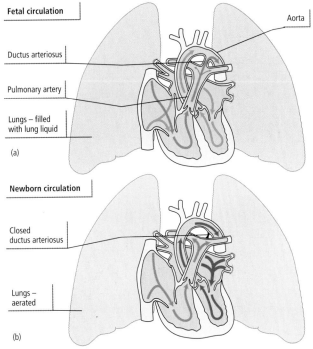

Fig. 11.1 Changes in the circulation at birth. (a) Fetal circulation. (b) Newborn circulation.

Physiologic changes in fetal–neonatal transition

- Before birth, the lungs are filled with fluid and oxygen is supplied by the placenta. The blood vessels that supply and drain the lungs are constricted (high pulmonary vascular resistance), so most blood from the right side of the heart bypasses the lungs and flows through the ductus arteriosus into the aorta (Fig. 11.1a).
- Shortly before and during labor, lung liquid production is reduced.
- During descent through the birth canal, the infant's chest is squeezed and some lung liquid exudes from the trachea.
- Multiple stimuli (thermal, chemical, tactile) initiate breathing. Serum cortisol, ADH (antidiuretic hormone), TSH (thyroid-stimulating hormone) and catecholamines dramatically increase.
- The first gasp is usually within a few seconds of birth. A high intrathoracic pressure is generated to achieve this. Most lung liquid is absorbed into the bloodstream or lymphatics within the first few minutes of birth.
- Aeration of the lungs is accompanied by increased arterial oxygen tension; the pulmonary artery blood flow increases and the pulmonary vascular resistance falls.
- Cord clamping removes the low-resistance placental circulation. This results in increased peripheral vascular resistance and an increase in systemic blood pressure.
- There is functional closure of the ductus arteriosus because of the fall in pulmonary vascular resistance and rise in systemic vascular resistance (Fig. 11.1b).

Abnormal transition from fetal to extrauterine life

The transition may be altered by a variety of antepartum or intrapartum events, resulting in cardiorespiratory depression, asphyxia or both (Table 11.1). The consequences may include hypoxic ischemic encephalopathy, persistent pulmonary hypertension and multi-organ system failure.

Table 11.1 Conditions associated with abnormal neonatal adaptation to extrauterine life.

Fetal	Maternal	Placental
Preterm/post-dates	General anesthetic	Chorioamnionitis
Multiple birth	Maternal drug therapy	Placenta previa
Forceps or vacuum-assisted delivery	Pregnancy-induced hypertension	Placental abruption
Breech or abnormal presentation	Chronic hypertension	Cord prolapse
Emergency cesarean section	Maternal infection	
Intrauterine growth restriction (IUGR)	Maternal diabetes mellitus	
Meconium-stained amniotic fluid	Polyhydramnios	
Abnormal fetal heart rate trace	Oligohydramnios	
Congenital malformations		
Anemia		
Infection		

The Apgar score

The Apgar score is used to describe an infant's condition during the first few minutes of life (Table 11.2). It is assigned at 1 and 5 minutes of life. If the score is still below 7 or the infant is requiring resuscitation, it is continued every 5 minutes until normal or 20 minutes of age.

Table 11.2 Apgar score.

| | Apgar score | | |
	0	1	2
Heart rate	Absent	Slow (<100 beats/minute)	>100 beats/minute
Respiration	Absent	Slow, irregular	Good, crying
Muscle tone	Limp	Some flexion of extremities	Active motion
Reflex irritability (response to stimulation)	No response	Grimace	Cough, sneeze, cry
Color	Blue or pale	Body pink, blue extremities	Pink

Key points

The Apgar score is not used to determine the need for resuscitation.

Evaluation for resuscitation is made second by second and is based on the three most important signs:
- respiration
- heart rate
- color.

Questions

How does resuscitation affect the Apgar score?

The Apgar score is assigned irrespective of resuscitation being performed.

Can one determine Apgar scores in preterm infants?

Yes. However, the extremely preterm infant's maximum score is reduced by poor muscle tone and weaker response to stimulation than term infants.

Asphyxia

With sustained, severe asphyxia (Fig. 11.2), a newborn infant will make increased respiratory effort, followed by a period of apnea (primary apnea). During primary apnea the heart rate falls but the blood pressure is maintained.

With continuing asphyxia, the infant starts to gasp and the heart rate falls. After several minutes, after a last gasp, there is secondary apnea. To recover, positive pressure ventilation is required.

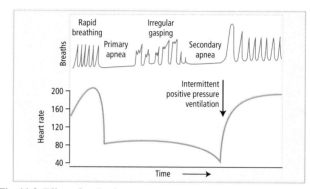

Fig. 11.2 Effect of asphyxia.

Question

What is the long-term significance of a low Apgar score (3 or less)?

An infant with a low Apgar score at 1 minute but responding rapidly to resuscitation has an excellent prognosis.

An infant with a low Apgar score beyond 10 minutes of age in spite of adequate resuscitation is at increasing risk of cerebral palsy the longer the score remains low.

Neonatal resuscitation is a rapid sequence of steps to be initiated if a baby's breathing or circulation is impaired (Fig. 12.1). The aim is to optimize the airway, breathing and circulation as quickly as possible.

Approximately 6–10% of all deliveries require some form of resuscitation. Ventilation, i.e. lung inflation, is the key. Only 0.1% of newborns of any gestation require chest compressions and medications during delivery room resuscitation.

Preparation

The presence of antepartum and intrapartum risk factors will usually allow the need for resuscitation to be anticipated. This enables health-care professionals skilled in neonatal resuscitation to be present. However, the need for neonatal resuscitation cannot always be predicted. All health-care professionals in maternity or neonatal units should be skilled in airway management, mask ventilation and cardiac compressions. Staff skilled in intubation and drug administration must be available at all times.

Before delivery

- Introduce yourself to the parents and explain why present.
- Review obstetric records.
- Wash hands and put on gloves.
- Turn on radiant warmer.

- Check equipment is present and functional:
  - clock
  - gas supply and delivery system (mask with T-piece connected to a pressure-limited circuit or bag and mask or Neopuff®)
  - airway adjuncts (Guerdel airway)
  - suction apparatus
  - laryngoscope, tracheal tube and introducer
  - stethoscope
  - venous access equipment and drugs.
- Warm towels available.

Specific questions to consider

- Will you need help?
- Is neonatal transport going to be needed?

Initial assessment at birth (Fig. 12.2)

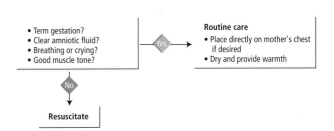

Fig. 12.2 Initial assessment at birth.

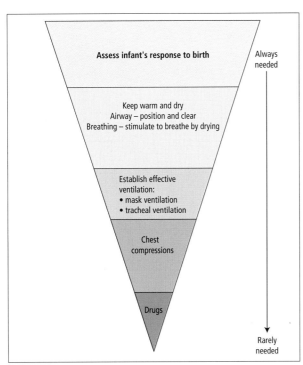

Fig. 12.1 Inverted pyramid showing relative frequency of procedures in neonatal resuscitation. (Adapted from *Textbook of Neonatal Resuscitation*, American Academy of Pediatrics/American Heart Foundation.)

Warmth/stimulation

Why important
Hypothermia may contribute to hypoglycemia, acidosis and even mortality, especially in VLBW (very low birthweight) infants.

Action
- Keep resuscitation area warm and draft-free.
- Perform resuscitation under radiant warmer.
- Dry infant, remove wet towel, then use dry towel.
- For extremely preterm infants, place infant in plastic wrapping with only head exposed.
- Stimulate if necessary – by drying with the towel. Flicking the soles of the feet can be used; do not inflict pain.

Key point

Do not allow newborn infants to get cold.

Although induced hypothermia is being studied in severely asphyxiated infants to decrease reperfusion injury, this is for specific indications under controlled conditions.

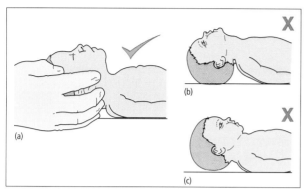

Fig. 12.3 Head position, the key to airway management. (a) Head in correct neutral position. (b) Head overextended – incorrect. (c) Head flexed – incorrect.

Airway

- **Position** – head in neutral position (Fig. 12.3), using towel beneath shoulders if desired, chin support (Fig. 12.4a) or jaw thrust (Fig. 12.4b).
- **Patency** – remove any meconium or blood if obstructing the airway. Not necessary to remove amniotic fluid.
- **Rare causes of airway obstruction** – choanal atresia, micrognathia (small jaw) or macroglossia (large tongue) – may require an oral airway.
- If cyanosed but breathing – **give oxygen**.

Breathing

Assessment

- Look for chest movement.
- Listen and feel for airflow.

Action

Initiate ventilation with a mask (Fig. 12.5) attached to a mechanical ventilator via a T-piece or a Neopuff® (provides pressure-limited oxygen) or a ventilation bag (Fig. 12.6) if:
- no or inadequate respiratory effort
- heart rate <100 beats/minute
- centrally cyanosed in spite of facial oxygen.

Mask ventilation

Begin mask ventilation with 100% oxygen for term infants. As this could potentially cause oxidant injury if <32 weeks' gestation, use air/oxygen blender to maintain oxygen saturation on pulse oximeter at 90–95%.

Inflation breaths

- Initially, for a term infant, give five breaths at an inflation pressure of 30–40 cm water for 2–3 seconds each. This will usually expand the

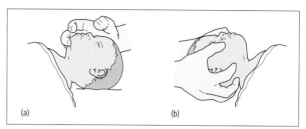

Fig. 12.4 (a) Chin support. (b) Jaw thrust.

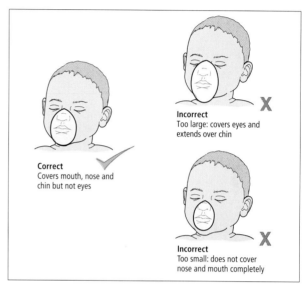

Fig. 12.5 Correct size and position of face mask. It should cover the mouth, nose and chin.

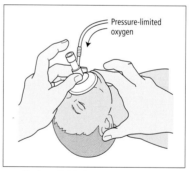

Fig. 12.6 Mask ventilation via T-piece connected to oxygen from a pressure-limited circuit, e.g. a mechanical ventilator or a Neopuff®.

lungs.
- Assess chest movement. If no chest movement recheck airway position and patency.

Ventilation breaths

- After inflation breaths, continue at 40–60 breaths/min. Use correct size mask and position, ventilating to see chest rise.
- Assess heart rate after 15–30 seconds.
- Stop when heart rate >100 breaths/minute and breathing effectively.

Intubation

Indications

- Mask ventilation ineffective (apnea or heart rate <100 beats/minute), i.e. after checking baby's head in neutral position, chin tilt/jaw thrust applied, longer inflation time given.
- Tracheal suction needed.
- Congenital upper airway abnormality.
- Prolonged ventilation needed.
- Extreme prematurity – delivery of surfactant.
  But:
- **Limit attempts to 20–30 seconds!**
- Mask-ventilate infant between attempts.

Circulation

- Assess heart rate with stethoscope or feel at the base of the umbilical cord.
- Initiate chest compressions (Fig. 12.7) if:
  - ventilation has been established **and** heart rate <60 beats/minute.

Key points

- Are the lungs inflated, i.e. good chest movement (and exhaled CO_2 detected, if measured)? If not, in neonates, chest compressions are ineffective.
- Call for help – giving chest compressions is easier with two people.

Drugs (Table 12.1)

Only use if no response in spite of:
- effective ventilation
- effective cardiac compression.

Key point

In neonates, drugs are useless unless ventilation is effective.

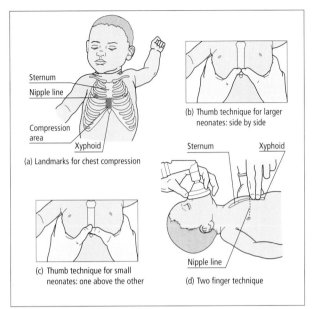

Sternum
Nipple line
Compression area
Xyphoid

(a) Landmarks for chest compression

(b) Thumb technique for larger neonates: side by side

Sternum   Xyphoid

(c) Thumb technique for small neonates: one above the other

Nipple line

(d) Two finger technique

Fig. 12.7 (a) Apply pressure to lower third of sternum, just below imaginary line joining the nipples. Avoid the xyphoid. Depress to reduce anteroposterior diameter of the chest by one-third (1–1.5 cm, ½ to ¾ inches) with no bounce. The thumb technique (b and c) is more effective than the two-finger technique and is recommended (d), but the two-finger technique is easier if you are alone or have small hands.

Give three compressions to one breath to achieve 90 compressions and 30 breaths (i.e. 120 events) in 1 minute. Stop and recheck heart rate every 30 seconds. Stop compressions when heart rate >60 beats per minute.

Special cases

Management of meconium

- If vigorous – no resuscitation needed.
- If depressed respirations – intubation and suction (using wall suction with a pressure-limiting device). Repeat intubation and suction as needed to clear airway. If heart rate slower than 60 beats/min start positive pressure ventilation.
- Monitor for subsequent respiratory distress.

Table 12.1 Drugs for neonatal resuscitation

Medication	Concentration	Dosage/route	Indications
Epinephrine (adrenaline)	1:10 000	IV: 0.1–0.3 mL/kg ET: 0.3–1 mL/kg	Heart rate <60 beats/minute after effective ventilation with 100% oxygen and chest compressions
Volume expander	Normal saline Whole blood	10 ml/kg IV	Suspected acute blood loss and/or signs of hypovolemia (poor perfusion, weak pulses, pallor)
Dextrose	10%	2.5 ml/kg (250 mg/kg) IV	Hypoglycemia
Sodium bicarbonate	0.5 mEq/ml (0.5 mmol/ml) (4.2% solution)	1–2 mEq/kg (1–2 mmol/kg) (2–4 ml/kg 4.2%) IV, slowly	Consider after prolonged arrest that does not respond to other therapy

Intravenous (IV) drugs are given via umbilical venous catheter or intraosseous route. Endotracheal (ET) delivery of epiphrine is easier but less reliable as absorption is variable. Consider ET route while IV access is obtained.

Failure to respond to resuscitation (Fig. 12.8)

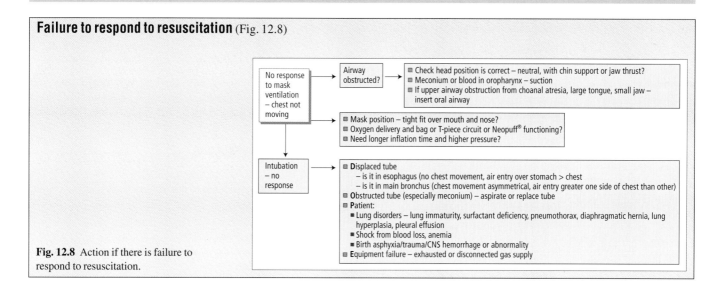

Fig. 12.8 Action if there is failure to respond to resuscitation.

Ethical decisions

International guidelines (2000) have been published for:
- non-initiation of resuscitation
  - infants less than 23 weeks of gestation (confirmed) or birthweight less than 400 g
  - anencephaly or trisomy 13 or 18 (confirmed)
- discontinuation of resuscitation
  - no heart beat or respiratory effort after 10 minutes of effective resuscitation.

Decisions need to be made about comfort care with parents and obstetric team.

This does not address the difficult ethical decisions concerning infants born at 23–25 weeks because of their:
- high mortality
- prolonged neonatal intensive care and hospitalization
- high risk of short-term morbidity and long-term disabilities
- high cost.

Parents will need information about mortality and morbidity, both national and local. Views will be affected by culture, religion and legal framework and may be limited by resources available. A center or country may have a birth weight or gestation cut off below which respiratory support is not provided.

Neonatal team will need to assess the situation at birth – whether gestation is correct, what is the infant's birthweight and condition. If in doubt, rather than hasty decisions in delivery room, often best to transfer to neonatal unit for detailed assessment. Disadvantage is that once intensive care initiated it may be difficult to withdraw treatment.

Overview (Fig. 12.9)

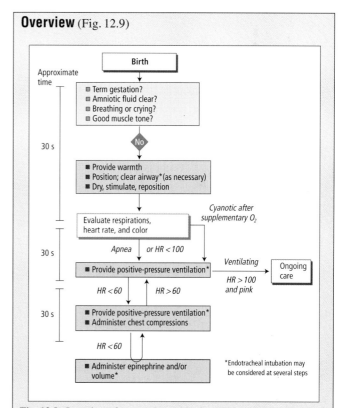

Fig. 12.9 Overview of neonatal resuscitation. (Adapted from *Neonatal Resuscitation*. American Academy of Pediatrics and American Heart Association, 2005.)

13 Hypoxic–ischemic encephalopathy

Asphyxia, from the Greek word meaning pulseless, is now used to mean a state in which gas exchange – placental or pulmonary – is compromised or ceases altogether, resulting in cardiorespiratory depression. Hypoxia, hypercarbia and metabolic acidosis follow. Compromised cardiac output diminishes tissue perfusion, causing hypoxic–ischemic injury to the brain and other organs. The neonatal condition is called hypoxic–ischemic encephalopathy (HIE) and is included as a cause of neonatal encephalopathy. In developed countries, approximately 0.5–1/1000 liveborn term infants develop HIE and 0.3/1000 have significant neurologic disability.

Hypoxic–ischemic brain injury may occur antepartum, during labor and delivery or postnatally (Fig. 13.1). As the term 'birth asphyxia' is imprecise and implies that the baby's condition is a consequence of birth, which may have medicolegal implications, it has been recommended that the term be discarded (*Guidelines for Perinatal Care*, American Academy of Pediatrics and American College of Obstetricians and Gynecologists, 2002). They have recommended using the term 'asphyxia' instead, but reserving it to describe an infant in whom all the following criteria are met:
- profound acidemia (pH <7) on an umbilical cord artery sample, if obtained
- Apgar score 0–3 for longer than 5 minutes
- neonatal neurologic manifestations, e.g. seizures, coma or hypotonia
- multisystem organ dysfunction.

Pathogenic mechanisms

These include:
- failure of gas exchange across the placenta – excessive or prolonged uterine contractions, placental abruption, ruptured uterus
- interruption of umbilical blood flow – cord compression including

shoulder dystocia, cord prolapse
- inadequate maternal placental perfusion, maternal hypotension or hypertension – often with intrauterine growth restriction (IUGR)
- compromised fetus – anemia, IUGR
- failure of cardiorespiratory adaptation at birth – failure to breathe (see Chapter 12).

Compensatory mechanisms

These include:
- diving reflex – redistribution of blood flow to vital organs (brain, heart and adrenals)
- sympathetic drive – increase in catecholamines, cortisol, antidiuretic hormone (ADH, vasopressin)
- utilization of lactate, pyruvate and ketones as an alternative energy source to glucose.

Neuronal death

Following a severe ischemic insult, some neuronal cells die rapidly (primary neuronal death). When the circulation is re-established, a sequence of biologic reactions may extend the zone of injury (secondary neuronal death). There is the potential to ameliorate this secondary damage (Fig. 13.2).

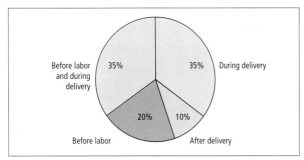

Fig. 13.1 Time of brain injury.

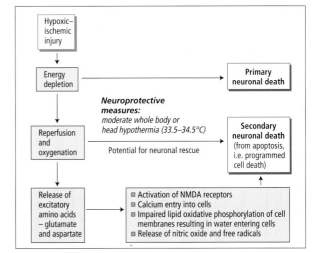

Fig. 13.2 Schematic diagram showing potential for prevention of secondary neuronal death.

Clinical manifestations

The clinical manifestations, investigations and management are summarized in Fig. 13.3.

Clinical staging of hypoxic–ischemic encephalopathy

This is done using a staging system, a sequential, systemic evaluation of the severity of brain injury. The most common is Sarnat (Table 13.1).

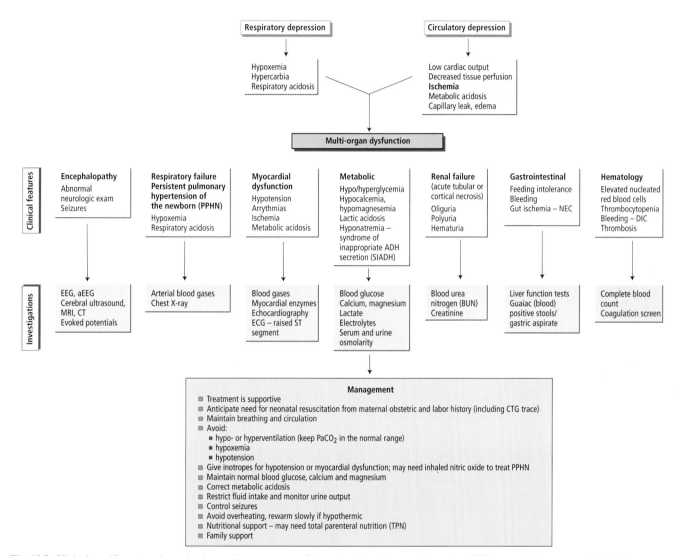

Fig. 13.3 Clinical manifestations, investigations and management of hypoxic–ischemic encephalopathy. (NEC – necrotizing enterocolitis; DIC – disseminated intravascular coagulation; EEG – electroencephalogram; aEEG – amplitude integrated EEG, cerebral function monitor; CTG – cardiotochography.)

Table 13.1 Sarnat staging of hypoxic–ischemic encephalopathy.

	Grade 1 (mild)	Grade 2 (moderate)	Grade 3 (severe)
Level of consciousness	Irritable/hyperalert	Lethargy	Coma
Muscle tone	Normal or hypertonia	Hypotonia	Flaccid
Tendon reflexes	Increased	Increased	Depressed or absent
Myoclonus	Present	Present	Absent
Seizures	Absent	Frequent	Frequent
Complex reflexes			
Suck	Active	Weak	Absent
Moro	Exaggerated	Incomplete	Absent
Grasp	Normal to exaggerated	Exaggerated	Absent
Oculocephalic (Doll's eye)	Normal	Overactive	Reduced or absent
Autonomic function			
Pupils	Dilated, reactive	Constricted, reactive	Variable or fixed
Respirations	Regular	Periodic	Ataxic, apneic
Heart rate	Normal or tachycardia	Bradycardia	Bradycardia
EEG	Normal	Low-voltage periodic or paroxysmal	Periodic or isoelectric
Prognosis	Good	Variable	High mortality and neurologic disability

Neuroimaging and functional studies (Table 13.2)

Table 13.2 Neuroimaging and functional studies and their indications and interpretation.

Procedure/test	Indication and interpretation
Standard	
EEG (electroencephalogram) or cerebral function monitor (Fig. 13.4) – best done as soon after birth as possible	Seizures. Background activity. Prognostic value
Cranial ultrasound	Easy to perform at bedside. Useful for defining normal anatomy and for evidence of prenatal injury on initial scan on admission. May detect cerebral edema, hyperechogenic basal ganglia, and abnormal blood flow velocity in middle and anterior cerebral arteries Useful for following sequence and timing of any changes
MRI scan	Imaging of choice in combination with ultrasound. Allows early recognition of bilateral basal ganglia injury, internal capsule, white matter and cortical injury, focal cerebral infarction, hemorrhage and malformations (Figs 13.5 and 13.6). However, an early scan on day 1–2 may appear normal
CT scan	For major malformation, hemorrhage, calcification, edema. Poor for posterior fossa, focal injury and myelin
BAER (brainstem auditory evoked responses)	Auditory nerve brainstem conduction
Not routinely available	
Positron emission tomography (PET)	Brain metabolic activity
Magnetic resonance spectroscopy:	
• Proton	Lactate and N-acetyl aspartate
• Phosphorus (seldom available)	Energy status of brain (Pi, ATP, ADP)
VEP (cortical visual evoked potentials)	Optic nerve – visual cortex pathway
Somatosensory evoked potentials	Median nerve – cortical responses, for prognosis

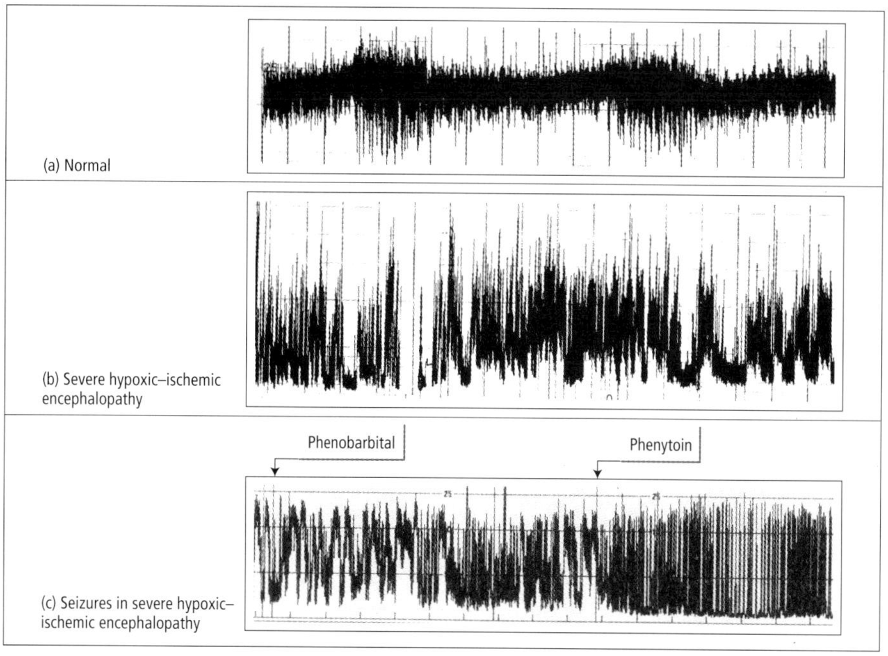

Fig. 13.4 Amplitude-integrated EEG (aEEG) trace from cerebral function monitor showing (a) normal term newborn – normal baseline (>5 mV); (b) severe hypoxic–ischemic encephalopathy – low baseline amplitude; (c) seizures in severe hypoxic–ischemic encephalopathy unresponsive to phenobarbital but responsive to phenytoin, although the trace remains abnormal. (Courtesy of Prof. Andrew Wilkinson.)

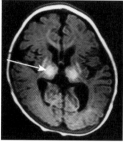

(a) Normal

(b) Severe hypoxic–ischemic encephalopathy

Phenobarbital   Phenytoin

(c) Seizures in severe hypoxic–ischemic encephalopathy

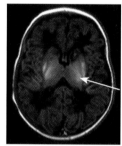

Fig. 13.5 MRI (axial TW1) at the level of the basal ganglia showing abnormal high signal in the posterolateral lentiform nuclei and thalami, loss of the normal high signal from myelin in the posterior limb of the internal capsule (arrow), abnormal signal in the head of the caudate nuclei and low signal throughout the white matter. These are typical of acute perinatal asphyxia in the first week after the insult. (Courtesy of Dr Frances Cowan.)

Fig. 13.6 MRI scan showing cerebral atrophy. Axial TW1 MRI at the level of the basal ganglia showing severe atrophy of the basal ganglia (arrow), thalami and white matter with enlarged ventricles and extracerebral space. There is also plagiocephaly. This degree of atrophy takes several weeks to develop. (Courtesy of Dr Frances Cowan.)

Outcome

In general:
- a normal neurologic exam and feeding well by 2 weeks of age suggest good prognosis
- mild HIE – usually normal outcome
- moderate – increased risk for motor and cognitive abnormalities, including cerebral palsy
- severe – mortality rate 75%, 80% of survivors will have neurologic sequelae.

The postnatal markers of poor prognosis are shown in Table 13.3.

Table 13.3 Postnatal markers of poor prognosis.

Persistence of clinical seizures

Persistently abnormal neurologic exam

Not feeding orally by 2 weeks of age

EEG with burst suppression or isoelectric pattern on any day or amplitude-integrated EEG (aEEG) with a low baseline amplitude

Abnormal EEG after day 12

Abnormal basal ganglia or marked brain atrophy on MRI

Alkaline intracellular pH or persistent tissue lactate on MR proton spectroscopy

Poor postnatal head growth

The incidence of severe birth injuries has fallen dramatically over the last 50 years. This is because prolonged, obstructed labor and difficult instrumental deliveries are avoided by cesarean section. However, birth injuries still occur, especially in infants who have had instrumental deliveries, shoulder dystocia, malpresentation (e.g. breech deliveries) or are preterm. They are usually classified according to their anatomic location.

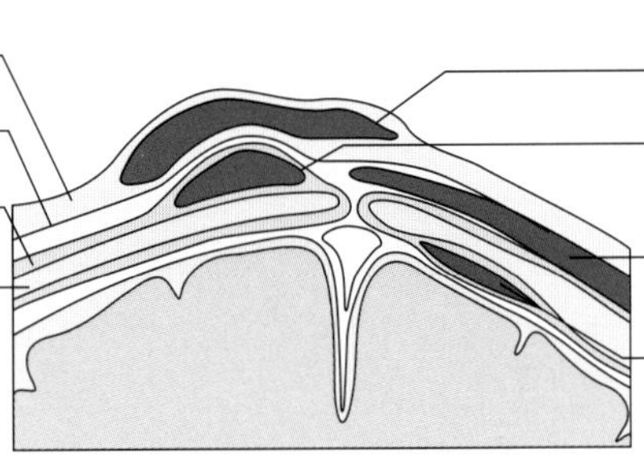

Fig. 14.1 Anatomic location of injuries to the head.

Common or important birth injuries

See Figure 14.1 and Table 14.1.

Table 14.1 Common or important birth injuries.

Lesion	Anatomic location	Comments	Clinical description and management
Injuries to the head			
Caput	Edema of the soft tissue of presenting part Crosses suture lines	Common and benign	Edema, bruising of scalp No treatment necessary; resolves in a few days Good prognosis
Chignon	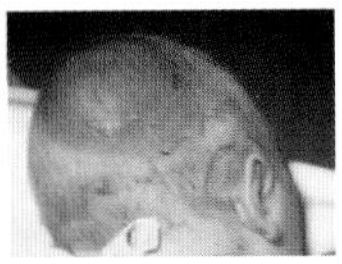 Over site of vacuum extraction	Less common since soft, flexible cups introduced	Edema, sometimes bruising, skin damage Resolves over several days
Cephalhematoma	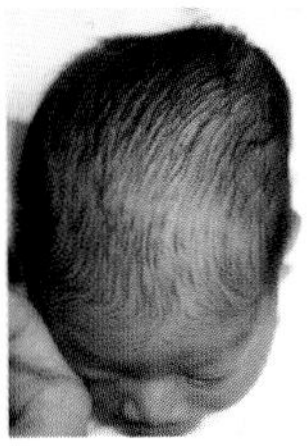 Subperiosteal Usually parietal Does not cross suture lines. May be bilateral	Relatively common Associated with prolonged or instrumental labor	Hematoma maximal on second day May be associated with skull fracture May calcify Exacerbates jaundice Resolves in days to months
Subgaleal (subaponeurotic) hemorrhage	Between galea aponeurosis and periosteum	Rare Risk factors: • prematurity • vacuum extraction May have underlying coagulopathy	Boggy appearance and pitting edema of scalp. Anterior displacement of the ears Prompt recognition is crucial as may rapidly progress to hypovolemic shock Transfusion of blood, fresh frozen plasma, coagulation factors
Skull fractures	Usually parietal bone; occipital in breech deliveries	Uncommon Usually forceps delivery, but also normal delivery	Soft tissue edema and cephalohematoma Fractures may be linear or depressed; latter may rarely require surgery Prognosis good
Minor injuries			
Forceps marks	From pressure of blades, especially rotational forceps	Less common as rotational forceps now seldom used	Bruising and/or skin abrasion Heals rapidly
Scalpel lacerations	Head or face	Scalpel incision at cesarean section	Usually small Depending on size and site, may need tapes to oppose edges, suturing, plastic surgical referral

Lesion	Anatomical location	Comments	Clinical description and management
Injuries to the face			
Facial palsy	Usually unilateral (right side in figure). If bilateral, suspect congenital cause	Pressure on maternal ischial spine or forceps delivery	Unilateral facial weakness on crying Eye remains open Resolves in 1–2 weeks If eye permanently open, use methylcellulose eye drops
Asymmetric crying facies		More common than facial palsy	In contrast to facial palsy, eye can close
Injuries to the neck and shoulders			
Fractured clavicle	Midclavicular area	Shoulder dystocia, breech. Snap may be heard during delivery	Edema, bruising, crepitation at the site; decreased active movement of arm Clavicular lump from callus formation during healing phase Confirm on X-ray Heals spontaneously
Brachial palsy Erb (> 90%) Nerves involved: C5, C6, ±C7		Shoulder dystocia, abnormal presentation, obstructed labor, macrosomia Phrenic nerve palsy – rare, diaphragm is elevated	Decreased shoulder abduction and external rotation, supination of wrist and finger extension (waiter's tip posture). Hand movement is preserved In 5% diaphragm palsy 90% resolve by 4 months To avoid contractures, perform passive range of motion ± splints Surgical referral if not recovered by 6 weeks
Klumpke (<1%) Nerves involved: C8, T1		Rare	Claw hand deformity from weakness of hand muscles and wrist flexors Horner syndrome in 30% (triad of dilated pupil, ptosis, i.e. drooping of eyelid, absent sweating)
Other injuries			
Extremities	Fracture of the humerus/femur	Breech, shoulder dystocia. May have underlying bone/ muscle disorder	Deformity, reduced movement of limb, pain on movement Orthopedic referral Splint to reduce pain. Rarely, hypovolemia from blood loss requires treatment Bones rapidly remodel
Spinal cord	Cervical, thoracic, lumbar spine	Rare. Instrumental delivery, may occur prenatally	Lack of movement below level of lesion Absent respiratory effort in high lesions Supportive care, steroids for spinal shock
Intra-abdominal organs	Ruptured liver, spleen	Macrosomia, breech, dystocia	Abdomen – distension, mass, discoloration, tenderness. Shock, pallor
	Renal injury Adrenal hemorrhage	Pre-existing hydronephrosis Prematurity, neuroblastoma	Hematuria Hypoglycemia, abdominal mass, coma, shock Intravascular volume support Abdominal ultrasound. Surgery unless bleed is contained (subcapsular hematoma)
Genitalia	Scrotum and labia majora	Breech	Bruising, hematoma Resolves

15 Routine care of the newborn infant

Most term infants start to breathe several seconds after birth and rapidly become pink and active. The umbilical cord is clamped and if the baby is breathing normally can be rapidly dried and handed directly to his/her mother. This will allow direct skin-to-skin contact, the baby being kept warm with a towel. Alternatively the baby can first be wrapped in warm towels. It is at this time that most babies are alert and are ready to begin to establish nursing at the breast.

Shortly after birth, the midwife, or pediatrician if attending the delivery, will examine the baby briefly to check there are no abnormalities. A more detailed examination, called the routine examination of the newborn, will be performed later, but within 24 hours of birth (see Chapter 16). Name tags will be attached to the baby and a record made to confirm that the baby passes urine and passes meconium within 24 hours of birth.

Routine care

Vitamin K
The administration of vitamin K as prophylaxis against hemorrhagic disease of the newborn should have been discussed with parents antenatally. It can be given either as a single, large dose by intramuscular injection, which provides reliable prevention but is an injection, or orally, which requires several doses to overcome its variable absorption, and protection is less reliable. Infants are at increased risk if they are breast-fed, as breast milk is low in vitamin K, if they have liver disease and if their mother is on anticonvulsant therapy.

Consent should be obtained before vitamin K is given.

Eye prophylaxis
In the US, all newborn infants are given erythromycin eye drops as prophylaxis against gonococcal and chlamydia eye infection. An alternative is silver nitrate eye drops, but this can cause chemical conjunctivitis and does not prevent chlamydial infection.

In the UK eye prophylaxis is not practiced, but gonococcal and chlamydia eye infection is extremely rare.

Circumcision
Widely performed in the US; only for religious reasons in the UK.

Appropriate analgesia should be provided for the procedure and postoperatively. May disrupt feeding and unsettle the infant for several days (see Chapter 50).

Meeting the family
Siblings, grandparents and other close family should be encouraged to visit to be introduced to the new member of the family.

Breast-feeding
Mothers often need considerable assistance and support to establish breast-feeding.

Umbilical cord care
Always wash hands before handling.
Keep dry and exposed to air.
Clean with water, avoid alcohol as it delays cord separation.
Fold diaper (nappy) below umbilicus.
In US, topical antibacterial agents (e.g. triple dye) widely used.

Emotions
Some mothers are emotionally labile during the first few days after birth. Even minor problems can cause considerable upset. Explanation and reassurance are required.

Mothers who develop postnatal depression or who are unable to care for their baby or have no suitable accommodation may be identified. Liaison with mental health or social services, voluntary services or health visitors and other community health professionals may be required.

Infants with disabilities or complex medical needs may require a multidisciplinary planning meeting before discharge. This is considered further in Chapter 68.

Screening

The use of a screening test depends on:
- prevalence of the disease
- ease with which the test can be performed
- false-positive and-false negative screening rate
- whether it significantly improves the prognosis
- cost.

Biochemical screening (called the Guthrie test in the UK)

This is performed on all infants. Blood spots, usually from a heel prick, are placed on a card which is sent to a reference laboratory.

In most centers in the US tandem mass spectometry is used to screen a wide range of disorders including:
- phenylketonuria (frequency 1:12 000)

Question

Can screening be performed for cystic fibrosis?
Yes, it can be performed, using the immunoreactive trypsin (IRT) test on the dried blood spot. The trypsin level is raised because of obstruction of the pancreatic ducts. It has a high false-positive rate, which can be reduced by combining it with DNA analysis.

There is some evidence that early diagnosis improves growth and cognitive development; there is the potential for better pulmonary outcomes. Screening is performed in some States and centers in the US; the Center for Disease Control and Prevention (CDC) has concluded that screening for cystic fibrosis is justified.

- hypothyroidism (1:4000).
- sickle cell disease
- thalassemia
- MCAD (medium chain acyl-CoA dehydrogenase) deficiency (1:10 000).

In the UK, screening is confined to the disorders listed above as well as for cystic fibrosis.

Audiology (see Chapter 60)

Neonatal hearing screening for all infants is being increasingly introduced. In some centers it is provided only for infants with risk factors, e.g. family history, hyperbilirubinemia requiring treatment or given potentially ototoxic drugs. All infants with preauricular tags or pits should have their hearing checked.

Other possible screening tests

Bilirubin at discharge

Suggested because of recent increase in kernicterus. Can identify infants at increased risk who require close monitoring at home. However, large number of tests are needed to identify small number of affected infants and its efficacy is unproven.

Pulse oximetry on all infants

Lower limb pulse oximetry to detect cyanotic congenital heart disease. However, low yield as prevalence is low.

Key points

In order to reduce the risk of SIDS, in addition to the key points shown in Fig. 15.1:
- Infant should sleep in own crib (cot), not in parents' bed, but in parents' bedroom.
- Infant should sleep on firm surface.
- Consider offering a pacifier (dummy) at nap time and bedtime (when >1 month old). (American Academy of Pediatrics, 2005.)

Routine hematocrit for polycythemia

Not recommended as not proven that treatment improves prognosis.

Health promotion

Parents should be provided with verbal and written advice about:
- feeding
- the importance of immunizations
- how to reduce the risk of SIDS (sudden infant death syndrome) (Fig. 15.1)
- the need for a car seat to take the baby home and whenever traveling in a car
- when to seek medical attention.

Discharge

Before discharge check that:
- feeding is being established successfully
- the nursing staff do not have concerns about the mother's handling of the baby
- the baby is well and not significantly jaundiced.

Question

Which immunizations should be given routinely in the immediate newborn period?

US
- Hepatitis B: initial dose recommended as part of universal immunization program and given before discharge.

UK
- BCG for TB: increasingly offered if living in high-risk area or for certain ethnic communities. Requires intradermal injection.
- Hepatitis B: given if mother is positive for hepatitis B surface antigen.

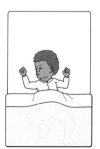

(a) Back to basics
Always put babies to sleep on their back (not prone or side)

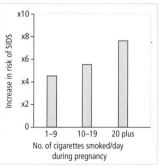

(b) Avoid smoking in your baby's presence

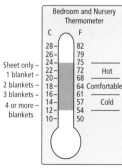

(c) Don't let your baby get too hot or cold

Fig. 15.1 Advice for parents to reduce the risk of SIDS. (Adapted from *Reduce the Risk of SIDS*. Department of Health, UK, 2001 and American Academy of Pediatrics, 2005.)

All babies are examined shortly after birth to check that transition to extrauterine life has proceeded smoothly and there are no major abnormalities. A comprehensive medical examination within 24 hours of birth, the 'routine examination of the newborn infant', should be performed.

The purpose is to:
- detect any abnormalities – a significant congenital anomaly is present at birth in 10–20 per 1000 live births
- confirm and/or consider the further management of any abnormalities detected antenatally
- consider potential problems related to maternal pregnancy history or familial disorders
- allow the parents to ask any questions and raise any concerns about their baby
- determine whether there is concern by caregivers about the care of the baby following discharge.
- provide health promotion, especially prevention of sudden infant death syndrome (SIDS) (see Chapter 15).

Preparation

Notes:
- Check maternal antenatal, labor and delivery notes.

Equipment:
- Tape measure.
- Stethoscope.
- Ophthalmoscope.

Environment:
- Warm room free from drafts.
- Privacy, suitably lit.
- Examine on firm mattress in crib
- Both parents present if possible.
- Always wash hands and clean stethoscope before each examination.

The infant

- The baby must be completely undressed during the course of the examination so that all the body is observed.
- Need a content, relaxed infant for successful examination.
- Examination is performed opportunistically, i.e. eyes when open, heart when quiet, hips left until last. However, the examination must be complete.

Developmental dysplasia of the hip, DDH (congenital dislocation of the hip, CDH)

Clinical examination:
- Performed on all infants – part of routine neonatal examination.
- Infant must be relaxed – if crying or kicking there is tightening of the muscles around the hip .
- There may be asymmetry of skin folds around the hip and shortening of the affected leg.
- Pelvis is stabilized with one hand; with the other, the examiner's middle finger is placed round the greater trochanter and the thumb around the distal medial femur.
- Both hips are fully abducted; full abduction may not be possible if the hip is dislocated.
- Check if dislocatable posteriorly (Barlow maneuver) (Fig. 16.2 (a)).
- Check if hip is dislocated and can be relocated into acetabulum (Ortolani maneuver) (Fig. 16.2(b)).

Risk increased:
- in female infants (9:1)
- if positive family history (20% of affected infants)
- if breech presentation (30% of affected infants)
- in infants with a neuromuscular disorder.

If abnormal or questionable clinical examination, arrange hip ultrasound at 4–6 weeks of age. Some centers perform hip ultrasound if there is a family history or breech delivery. Role of routine ultrasound screening of all infants still being assessed – can identify some missed on clinical examination and some with shallow acetabular shelf not detectable on clinical examination, but has appreciable false-positive rate (7%) and is expensive.

For management see Chapter 59.

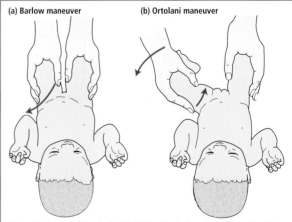

(a) Test for dislocatable hip. The hip is held flexed and adducted. The femoral head is pushed downwards. If dislocatable, the femoral head will be pushed posteriorly out of the acetabulum
(b) Test for dislocated hip. Abduct hip with upward leverage of femur. A dislocated hip will return with a palpable **clunk** into the acetabulum

Fig. 16.1 Barlow and Ortolani maneuvers.

Routine examination of newborn infants (Table 16.1, Figs 16.2 and 16.3)

Table 16.1 Significant congenital abnormalities which may be identified on routine examination.

Dysmorphic infant (see Chapter 8)

Cataracts (see Chapter 60)

Cleft lip and palate (see Chapter 56)

Heart murmurs (see Chapter 47)

Urogenital – hypospadias, undescended testes (see Chapter 50)

DDH (developmental dysplasia of the hip)

Imperforate anus (see Chapter 46)

Spinal anomalies (see Chapter 57)

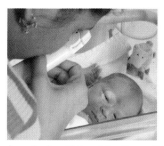

Fig. 16.2 Checking for red reflex. If absent, i.e. the pupil is white (cataracts, glaucoma, retinoblastoma), refer directly to an ophthalmologist. Also check eye looks normal, e.g. for a coloboma, a key-shaped defect in the iris.

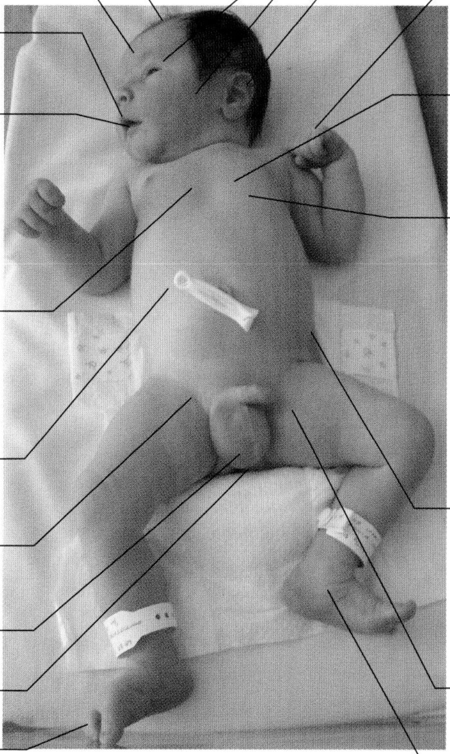

General appearance, posture, movements – are they normal?

Fontanelle and skull structures feel normal

Facies – any dysmorphic features e.g. Trisomy 21 (Down syndrome)

Palate – inspect and palpate to identify cleft palate

Cyanosis of tongue – if in doubt check oxygen saturation with pulse oximeter

Breathing and chest wall movement – observe for respiratory distress:
- increased respiratory rate
- flaring of nostrils
- grunting
- chest retractions (sternal and intercostal)

Abdomen:
- normal liver 1–2cm below costal margin, spleen tip and left kidney may be palpable
- any masses – investigate with ultrasound

Hips – check for developmental dysplasia of the hips (see opposite)

Genitalia – check testes in scrotum and normal penis in boys and normal anatomy in girls

Anus – check patency

Feet – check for talipes

Eyes – check with ophthalmoscope for red reflex

Plethora or pale? If suspected, check hematocrit

Ears – low-set, malformed or preauricular tags/pits?

Hands – check for extra digits, palmar creases

Jaundice – if present in first 24 hours, needs investigation

Heart – auscultate. Normal heart rate 110–160 beats/min but may drop to 80 beats/min during sleep
Heart murmur – see Chapter 47

Back and spine: check from top to bottom. Sacral dimples below the line of the natal cleft – common and benign. If proximal to natal cleft, ultrasound to identify if there is a track to the spinal cord, though rare. Check the back for a tuft of hair, swelling, nevus or other lesion over the spine, which may indicate vertebral or spinal cord abnormality, e.g. spina bifida occulta or tethered cord. If present, arrange ultrasound, but MRI scan may be required

Femoral pulses:
- reduced in coarctation of the aorta. If suspected, check by measuring blood pressure in all four limbs. Difference > 15mmHg is significant
- bounding in patent ductus arteriosus

Muscle tone:
- observe for normal movements of limbs
- feel when handling the baby (support the head when picking up baby)
- on holding prone, term babies will lift their head to horizontal position

Measurements (at 40 weeks):

	50th centile	(10th–90th centile)	Comments
Birth weight	3.5 kg	(2.8–4.5 kg)	
Head circumference	35 cm	(33.5–37 cm)	Maximal occipito-frontal diameter
Length	51 cm	(48–53.5 cm)	Routinely measured in USA, not in UK Inaccurate unless hips and knees are straightened

Fig. 16.3 Routine examination of newborn infants.

The newborn infant's neurologic development progresses markedly with gestational age. This needs to be taken into account when performing a neurologic examination, and also accounts for many of the components of the neurologic examination also being used in the clinical assessment of gestational age (Ballard or Dubowitz score; see Chapter 77).

A detailed neurologic examination is performed if there are any concerns about neurologic abnormality. A normal neurologic exam is helpful prognostically. Following hypoxic–ischemic encephalopathy, a normal neurologic examination and normal feeding by 2 weeks of age are associated with a good prognosis. Very low birthweight infants with a normal neurologic examination and intracranial ultrasound at 40 weeks are highly unlikely to develop significant motor disability and the predictive value of combined assessment is better than ultrasound alone.

The neurologic development described here is adapted from that described by Amiel-Tison, who has also devised a standardized examination with 10 components.

States of alertness

An infant's state of alertness can be classified (Prechtl scale):
- State 1: Eyes closed, regular respiration, no movements
- State 2: Eyes closed, irregular respiration, no gross movements
- State 3: Eyes open, no gross movements,
- State 4: Eyes open, gross movements, no crying
- State 5: Eyes open or closed, crying

For satisfactory neurologic assessment infants need to be in state 3, when they are quiet but alert, i.e. able to fix and follow. However, the clinician may have to bring the baby to this state. Inability to do this may occur because the infant is abnormally lethargic or hyperexcitable (or deeply asleep or hungry!). An abnormal cry may also indicate abnormal neurology.

Visual fixing and following

A normal term infant should make eye-to-eye contact when held about 30 cm from the observer. The infant will fix and follow a face or red ball moving from side to side.

Hearing

Infants respond to noise with a facial grimace, turning of the head or startle.

Consolability

This is the response of the crying infant to a voice or soothing movements, such as rocking from side to side. It indicates communication between the infant and caregiver.

Head circumference

This is a surrogate measure of head volume and subsequently of head growth.

Face (cranial nerves)

There should be normal facial movements, blinking of the eyes and ability to suck strongly.

Posture and spontaneous motor activity

Posture

Posture at term is flexed (Fig. 17.1). Movements are smooth, symmetric and varied. The infant can move the fingers and can abduct the thumbs.

Passive tone in limbs and trunk

Develops from hypotonia at 24 weeks of gestation to strong flexor tone at 40 weeks, initially in the lower then upper limbs (Fig. 17.2).

Active tone in limbs and trunk

See Fig. 17.3.

32 weeks	40 weeks
Arms extended Some flexion of the legs	Full flexion of all four limbs

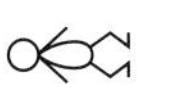

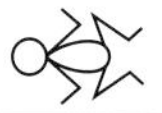

Fig. 17.1 Posture.

Popliteal angle		Foot dorsiflexion		Scarf sign	
With thigh beside abdomen, extend knee as far as possible		With knee flexed, ankle is dorsiflexed Measure angle between dorsum of foot and anterior of leg		Hand pulled across chest towards opposite shoulder Position of elbow noted	
32 weeks	Term	32 weeks	Term	32 weeks	Term
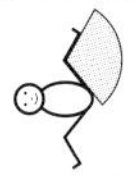	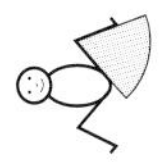	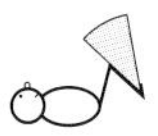	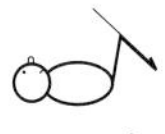	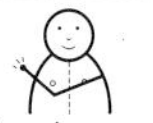 Largely passes midline	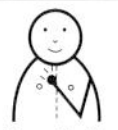 Very tight
120°–110°	90° or less	40°–30°	0°	Very weak resistance	Does not reach midline

Fig. 17.2 Passive tone in limbs and trunk.

Primary reflexes

Primary or primitive reflexes reflect brainstem activity (Fig. 17.4). They are a manifestation of central nervous system programming with later suppression by higher cortical function. If they cannot be elicited, suggests central nervous system depression. More important, their persistence suggests damage to upper cortical control (Table 17.1).

Deep tendon reflexes

May be depressed with lower motor neuron lesions, occasionally increased with upper motor neuron lesions. May reveal asymmetry. Ankle clonus is common and usually of no pathologic significance.

Plantar responses

Elicited by stroking the lateral part of the foot from heel to toe. Unhelpful at this age as normal response may be flexor (toe down) or extensor (toe up).

Righting reaction		Neck flexor tone (raise to sit)		Ventral suspension	
Holding infant upright under axillae		Holding infant's shoulders, pull from lying to sitting			
32 weeks	40 weeks	32 weeks	40 weeks	32 weeks	40 weeks
Brief support of lower limbs only	Upright and takes weight for few secs	No movement of head forwards	Minimal head lag. Similarly for neck extensor tone (back to lying)	Some extension of head and back	Head extended above body, back extended and limbs fully flexed

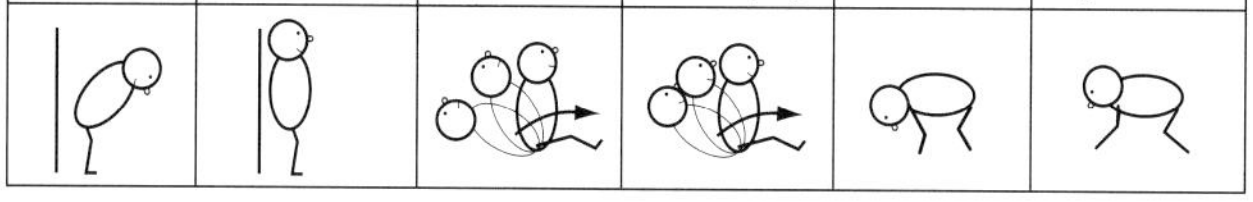

Fig. 17.3 Active tone in limbs and trunk.

Table 17.1 Primary reflexes.

Reflex	Disappearance (corrected age)
Placing	3 months
Palmar grasp	3 months
Plantar grasp	3 months
Moro	4 months
Asymmetric tonic neck reflex (ATNR)	6 months

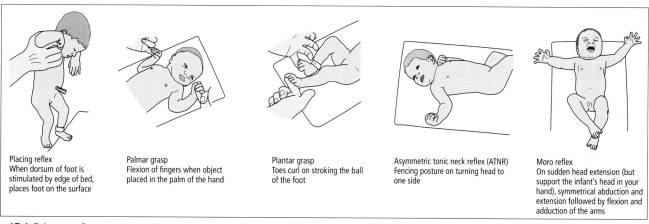

Placing reflex
When dorsum of foot is stimulated by edge of bed, places foot on the surface

Palmar grasp
Flexion of fingers when object placed in the palm of the hand

Plantar grasp
Toes curl on stroking the ball of the foot

Asymmetric tonic neck reflex (ATNR)
Fencing posture on turning head to one side

Moro reflex
On sudden head extension (but support the infant's head in your hand), symmetrical abduction and extension followed by flexion and adduction of the arms

Fig. 17.4 Primary reflexes.

The family must, of course, be included in the care of all newborn infants, whether well or critically ill. The birth of a healthy newborn infant is usually a joyous occasion fulfilling the dreams and hopes of the parents. If the baby is extremely premature, sick, has malfor-mations or dies, these dreams will be shattered and the family will experience considerable distress. The family will need sensitive assessment, discussion and support. How this is done will influence their ability to cope and recover in the short and long term.

Attachment

What is maternal attachment?

It is the intense relationship which develops between a mother and her child, providing protection and nurturing for the child (Fig. 18.1).

In many animals, e.g. ducks or penguins, there is a critical, sen-sitive period for mother–infant bonding immediately after birth, when the mother and her offspring must be in direct contact. If this does not happen the mother fails to recognize that the newborn is hers. Attachment in humans does not necessarily happen instantly, but develops over time. Although touching and nursing the baby shortly after birth is helpful in promoting attachment, and should be encouraged, humans can still become attached to their infants where this does not occur, for example if the infant is admitted directly to the neonatal unit.

Fathers and other family members also develop attachment with the newborn baby.

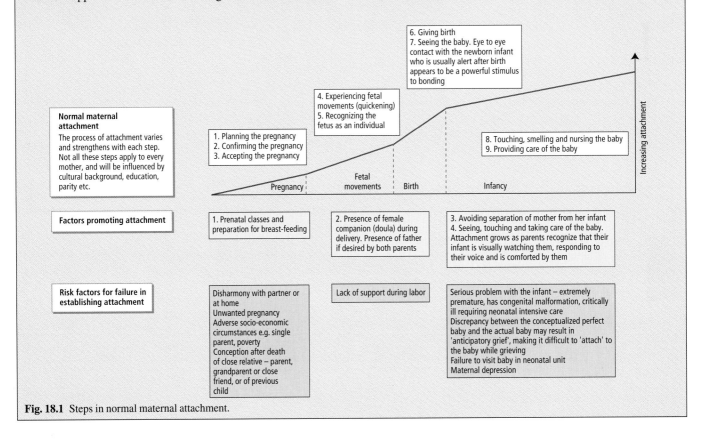

Fig. 18.1 Steps in normal maternal attachment.

Communicating with parents

Parents and family want open communication about their baby. Professionals need to provide not only accurate and realistic information about the baby's problems but to also listen to and address the family's anxieties and feelings. The needs of each of the family members should be elicited, as they may differ. Some specific circumstances regarding communicating with parents related to perinatal care are considered below.

Antenatal identification of fetal abnormality or potential abnormality

- Many problems, including major malformations and preterm delivery, are now identified before birth. The recognition of many minor malformations or the possibility of an abnormal finding in the fetus has become a common cause of additional anxiety for parents.
- The neonatal team should be involved and present a realistic picture. First discuss the positive aspects and tend towards optimism – describe a glass as half full rather than half empty. Facts should be disclosed but unsubstantiated fears not shared with the family.
- Problems should be anticipated and their consequences and management discussed with the family. If appropriate, a tour of the neonatal intensive care unit (NICU) before delivery should be conducted.

Admission of the infant to the neonatal unit

See Chapter 22.

Infants with serious congenital malformations

The crisis of the birth of a child with a serious malformation can result in emotional turmoil, the parents mourning the loss of the normal child they expected whilst also needing to become attached to their living but abnormal child. Doctors and other health professionals will need to explain the nature and implications of the disorder to the parents and family and may need to provide considerable emotional support to help families in this difficult situation (Table 18.1).

Table 18.1 How parents wish to be told the diagnosis of a serious problem or life-threatening illness.

Setting	**Explain long-term prognosis**
In private and comfort	If child is likely to die, listen to concerns about time, place and nature of death
Uninterrupted	Outline the support/treatment available
Unhurried	
Both parents (or friend/relative) present if possible	**Address feelings**
Senior doctor	Be prepared to tolerate reactions of shock, especially anger or weeping
Nurse or social worker present	Acknowledge uncertainty
Translator if necessary	How is it likely to affect the family?
Some families find it helpful to have a tape recording of the interview or to take notes	What and how to tell other children, relatives and friends?
	Concluding the interview
Establish contact	Elicit what parents have understood
Find out what the family knows or suspects	Clarify and repeat, particularly highlighting immediate situation and next steps
Respect family's vulnerability	Acknowledge that it may be difficult for parents to absorb all the information
Use the child's name	Mention sources of support
Do not avoid looking at them	Give parents a contact telephone number
Be direct, open, sympathetic	Give address of self-help group
Provide information	**Follow-up**
Flexibility is essential	Offer early follow-up and arrange date
Pace rather than protect from bad news. Some families want a lot of information at once, others prefer shorter interviews more often	Suggest to families that they write down questions in preparation for next appointment
Name the illness or condition	Ensure adequate communication of content of interview to other members of staff, family practitioner and health visitor and other professionals, e.g. a referring pediatrician
Describe symptoms relevant to child's condition	
Discuss etiology – parents will usually want to know	
Anticipate and answer questions. Don't avoid difficult issues because parents have not thought to ask	

(Adapted from Woolley H, Stein A, Forrest GC, Baum JD. Imparting the diagnosis of life threatening illness in children. *Br Med J* 1989; **298**: 1623–6)

19 Feeding

Human milk is recommended as the exclusive food for all term infants for the first 6 months of life. Thereafter, weaning with solid foods is commenced. Human milk is also recommended for preterm infants but may need fortification. All mothers should be encouraged and supported to breast-feed. Counseling should commence early in pregnancy and mothers should be assisted by nursing or lactation specialists.

The choice to breast- or bottle-feed is personal and formula feeding should not be criticized.

Nutritional characteristics of human milk compared with unmodified cow's milk

Protein

- Low protein content (whey:casein, 60:40) – more easily digestible.
- High free amino acids and urea; glutamine, the predominant amino acid, stimulates enterotropic hormones, enhancing feeding tolerance.

Fat

- Unsaturated.
- Contains long-chain polyunsaturated fatty acids (LCPUFAs) – needed for nervous system development (now incorporated into formula, as is arachidonic acid, ARA).

Carbohydrate

- High lactose.

Minerals

- Low renal solute load.
- Reduced phosphate:calcium ratio.

Vitamins

Supplementation required to breast milk to meet daily requirements.

Formula

Formula is humanized, i.e. manipulated to resemble human milk. However, there are still differences in amino acid and fatty acid composition and it does not contain the anti-infective properties of human milk. In developing countries, infection from reconstituting milk powder with contaminated water is a major health problem.

Unmodified cow's, goat's and sheep's milks are unsuitable for infants. Soy formula is sometimes used to prevent allergic disorders such as eczema and asthma, although evidence for this is lacking. About 10–30% of infants with cow's milk protein intolerance become sensitive to soy.

Steps to successful breast-feeding

- Place the infant on the breast either immediately or soon after birth.
- Provide quiet, supportive environment with comfortable positioning (Fig. 19.1).
- Demand feeding is preferable to a fixed schedule. This stimulates milk production and reduces feeling of fullness and discomfort. May be put to the breast 8–12 or more times per 24 hours.
- Put to both breasts at each feeding. Switch sides when baby pauses and lets go of breast. Allow unrestricted duration of feeds. Begin each feeding with the breast last nursed from.
- Emptying the breast adequately avoids engorgement.

- Initial milk is colostrum – low in volume, high in protein and immunoglobulin content. Takes 24–72 hours for breast milk to come in.
- Warn mothers that babies initially lose weight (up to 10% of birth weight) and only put on weight after day 4 of life. They should be back to birth weight by 10–21 days.
- Do not give supplementary water or formula unless medically indicated.
- Allow mothers and infants to stay together (rooming-in) 24 hours a day.
- Inform mothers of breast-feeding support groups.

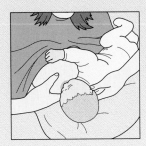
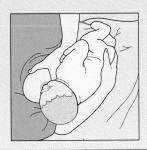
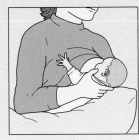

Fig. 19.1 Positioning for breast-feeding. (Adapted from UNICEF UK Baby Friendly Initiative.)

Breast-feeding

Advantages of breast-feeding for the infant

Immediate:

- Promotes mother–infant bonding.
- Ideal nutritional composition (see below).
- Contains immune factors (e.g. secretory IgA).
- Reduces gastroenteritis, possibly other infections.
- Less feeding intolerance.
- Reduces incidence of necrotizing enterocolitis in preterm infants.
- Promotes ketone production as an alternative energy substrate to glucose in first few days of life.

Long term:

- May decrease incidence and severity of eczema and asthma, but evidence is conflicting.
- Less obesity, insulin-dependent diabetes mellitus (type 1) and inflammatory bowel diseases (Crohn disease and ulcerative colitis).
- IQ (intelligence quotient) is increased 6–8 points if breast-fed.

Advantages of breast-feeding for the mother

- Enhances mother–infant bonding.
- More rapid postpartum weight loss.
- Decreased risk of osteoporosis.
- Decreased risk of breast and ovarian cancer.
- Increases time between pregnancies, which is important in developing countries.

Complications/disadvantages of breast-feeding for the infant

- Cannot tell how much milk the baby has taken. This is monitored by checking baby's weight, initially every few days, then less often.
- Dehydration may occur if:
  - inadequate milk supply/poor feeding technique
  - hot weather.
- Jaundice associated with breast milk:
  - common
  - exacerbated by dehydration
  - even if requiring phototherapy, breast-feeding should not be discontinued
  - is prolonged (>2 weeks of age) in 15% – will require investigations to be performed.
- Multiple births:
  - twins can often be breast-fed (Fig. 19.2), but rarely higher-order births.

Key point

'Breast is best' for feeding newborn infants.

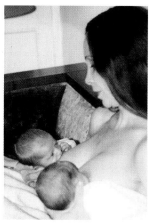

Fig. 19.2 Successful breast-feeding of twins.

- Vitamin K:
  - low level in breast milk may predispose to hemorrhagic disease of the newborn
  - prophylaxis is required.

Complications/disadvantages of breast-feeding for the mother

- Maternal feeling of inadequacy/upset if unsuccessful.
- Breast engorgement, cracked nipples – may be helped by manual expression or breast pump.
- Mastitis – requires maternal treatment and may disrupt feeding.

Contraindications to breast-feeding

- **Maternal HIV** – breast-feeding contraindicated in developed countries but advised in developing countries if no safe alternative is available.
- **Maternal TB** infection (active).
- **Inborn errors of metabolism** – galactosemia, phenylketonuria.

Drugs in breast milk

- Most drugs are excreted in breast milk in such small quantities they do not affect the infant.
- Where possible, all drugs, including self-medication, should be avoided during breast-feeding. Most mothers who need medications can continue breast-feeding, but a few drugs preclude breast-feeding:
  - cytotoxic agents, e.g. methotrexate and cyclophosphamide
  - radioactive iodine.

  Check a formulary.

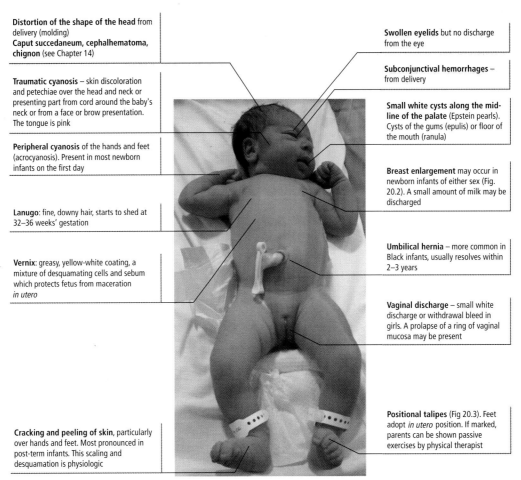

Distortion of the shape of the head from delivery (molding)
Caput succedaneum, cephalhematoma, chignon (see Chapter 14)

Traumatic cyanosis – skin discoloration and petechiae over the head and neck or presenting part from cord around the baby's neck or from a face or brow presentation. The tongue is pink

Peripheral cyanosis of the hands and feet (acrocyanosis). Present in most newborn infants on the first day

Lanugo: fine, downy hair, starts to shed at 32–36 weeks' gestation

Vernix: greasy, yellow-white coating, a mixture of desquamating cells and sebum which protects fetus from maceration *in utero*

Cracking and peeling of skin, particularly over hands and feet. Most pronounced in post-term infants. This scaling and desquamation is physiologic

Swollen eyelids but no discharge from the eye

Subconjunctival hemorrhages – from delivery

Small white cysts along the midline of the palate (Epstein pearls). Cysts of the gums (epulis) or floor of the mouth (ranula)

Breast enlargement may occur in newborn infants of either sex (Fig. 20.2). A small amount of milk may be discharged

Umbilical hernia – more common in Black infants, usually resolves within 2–3 years

Vaginal discharge – small white discharge or withdrawal bleed in girls. A prolapse of a ring of vaginal mucosa may be present

Positional talipes (Fig 20.3). Feet adopt *in utero* position. If marked, parents can be shown passive exercises by physical therapist

Fig. 20.1 Transient abnormalities in the first few days of life.

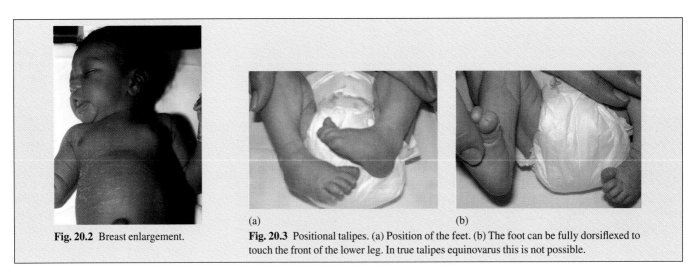

(a)   (b)

Fig. 20.2 Breast enlargement.

Fig. 20.3 Positional talipes. (a) Position of the feet. (b) The foot can be fully dorsiflexed to touch the front of the lower leg. In true talipes equinovarus this is not possible.

Skin lesions

Stork bites

Pink macules on upper eyelids, mid-forehead (also called salmon patch) and nape of the neck (Fig. 20.4). Common. Dilated superficial capillaries. Those on the eyelids and forehead fade over the first year. Those on the neck persist but are covered with hair.

Milia

White, pinhead-sized pimples on the nose and cheeks and forehead. Resolve during first month of life. Are from retention of keratin and sebaceous material in the pilosebaceous follicles.

Miliaria

Pin-sized vesicles, particularly over the neck and chest. Usually develop at 2–3 weeks. Caused by sweat that is retained due to obstructed eccrine glands. Avoid excessive clothing and heating.

Erythema toxicum

Small, firm, white or yellow pustules on erythematous base (Fig. 20.5). It is the most common transient lesion, usually appears at 1–3 days but up to 2 weeks of age; primarily on trunk, extremities and perineum. Moves to different sites within hours. Contains eosinophils. May be present at birth.

Mongolian blue spots

Blue–black macular discoloration at base of the spine and on the buttocks (Fig. 20.6). Usually but not invariably in Black or Asian infants. Sometimes also on the legs and other parts of the body. Fade slowly over the first few years. Of no significance unless misdiagnosed as bruises.

Transient pustular melanosis (transient neonatal pustulosis)

Resembles miliaria, but present at birth and may continue to appear for several weeks. Superficial vesiculo-pustular lesions rupture within 48 hours to leave small pigmented macules with white surround. More common in Black infants, in whom the lesions are often hyperpigmented.

Harlequin color change

Sharply demarcated blanching down one half of the body – one side of the body red while the other is pale. Lasts a few minutes. Thought to be due to vasomotor instability. It is benign.

Sucking blisters

Vesicles on hand, fingers, or lips, from vigorous sucking *in utero*.

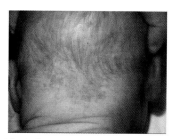

Fig. 20.4 Stork bite (salmon patch).

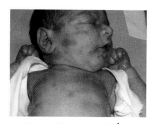

Fig. 20.5 Erythema toxicum. (Courtesy of Dr Nim Subhedar.)

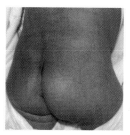

Fig. 20.6 Mongolian blue spot.

Other minor abnormalities (Figs 20.7–9)

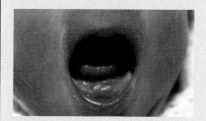

Fig. 20.7 Natal teeth. Front lower incisors present at birth. Remove if loose to avoid the risk of aspiration.

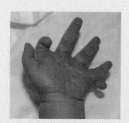

Fig. 20.8 Extra digits. Usually connected by a skin tag but may contain bone. Common anomaly – often hereditary. Consult plastic surgeon. Tying with silk thread may leave residual neuroma.

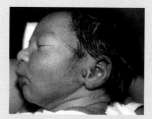

Fig. 20.9 Ear tags. Consult plastic surgeon. Check that the ear and hearing is normal. If there is an ear anomaly, some centers ultrasound the kidneys as slight increased risk of renal abnormalities.

Anticipation

Many neonatal problems can be anticipated or prevented by awareness of conditions that are detected antenatally (Tables 21.1 and 21.2) or which develop during labor or delivery (Table 21.3). This necessitates close liaison between the health professionals caring for the mother and fetus and the pediatricians. Some common examples which may be anticipated developing in the neonatal period are listed below. They are described in more detail in the relevant chapters.

Maternal or antenatal conditions (Table 21.1)

Table 21.1 Neonatal problems associated with maternal conditions.

Maternal medical condition	Neonatal problem
Diabetes mellitus	Neonatal hypoglycemia Polycythemia Jaundice Congenital malformations
Maternal hyperthyroidism	Neonatal hyperthyroidism or hypothyroidism from maternal drug treatment
Autoimmune thrombocytopenia	Neonatal thrombocytopenia
SLE (systemic lupus erythematosus)	Heart block, rash
Red blood cell isoimmunization Rhesus and other red cell antibodies. ABO incompatibility (mother group O, infant A or B)	Jaundice, anemia
Blood tests Hepatitis B positive HIV infection Syphilis serology positive	Immunization ± prophylaxis Preventative therapy, advice about breast-feeding Treatment if necessary
Abnormal ultrasound Renal (commonest) e.g. hydronephrosis Cardiac Other abnormalities	May need prophylactic antibiotics, ultrasound and VCUG (vesicocystourethrogram) Echocardiography – liaise with pediatric cardiologist involved antenatally Management as planned antenatally
Cervical smear (in US) Gonococcus or *Chlamydia trachomatis*	Check for conjunctivitis
Maternal drugs Drug abuse Alcohol	Neonatal drug withdrawal Fetal alcohol syndrome
Prolonged rupture of membranes Chorioamnionitis Maternal fever >38°C Maternal group B streptococcal bacteriuria or colonization	Neonatal infection

Fetal conditions (Table 21.2)

Table 21.2 Neonatal problems associated with fetal conditions.

Fetal condition	Neonatal problem
Intrauterine growth restriction (IUGR) or large for gestational age	Hypoglycemia Polycythemia
Multiple births	Anemia/polycythemia Twin–twin transfusion syndrome Congenital malformations Intrauterine growth restriction (IUGR)

Labor and delivery (Table 21.3)

Table 21.3 Neonatal problems associated with abnormal labor and delivery.

Labor and delivery	Neonatal problem
Antepartum hemorrhage	Hypoxic–ischemic encephalopathy, anemia
Markedly abnormal CTG trace	Hypoxic–ischemic encephalopathy
Cesarean section	TTNB (transient tachypnea of the newborn)
Instrumental delivery Vacuum extraction	Chignon, jaundice Localized bruising Cephalhematoma, jaundice Subgaleal (subaponeurotic) hemorrhage – anemia, shock
Forceps	Facial palsy
Breech position	DDH (developmental dysplasia of the hip) Birth injuries Hypoxic–ischemic encephalopathy
Shoulder dystocia	Hypoxic–ischemic encephalopathy Erb palsy Fractured clavicle or humerus
Meconium	Meconium aspiration
Need for prolonged resuscitation at delivery	Hypoxic–ischemic encephalopathy

Overview of common medical problems

Most newborn infants are healthy, but may develop some of the clinical features described below. Differentiating the clinically significant from the transient and benign can be difficult. An approach to these problems is given in Fig. 21.1. For details see specific chapters.

Conjunctivitis
Sticky eyes – common
Clean with sterile (boiled) water
If conjunctivitis purulent or eyelids red and swollen, exclude bacterial cause including gonococcus and chlamydia

Vomiting
Babies often vomit milk. If persistent or bile stained may be from intestinal obstruction. If it contains blood, malrotation must be excluded, but is usually swallowed maternal blood from delivery or maternal breast
Abdominal distension may be from lower intestinal obstruction

Poor feeding
Usually related to problems in establishing breast-feeding
However, can be presentation of:
- Infection
- Hypoglycemia
- Electrolyte disturbance
- Inborn error of metabolism

Cyanotic/dusky spells
Normal infants sometimes become dusky or cyanosed around the mouth, often during feeds, in the first few days.
Conditions which need to be excluded are:
- Cyanotic congenital heart disease
- Polycythemia
- Infection

Mucus
Many babies produce a considerable amount of mucus on the first day. This needs to be differentiated from the infant with esophageal atresia who is unable to swallow saliva, which pools in the mouth

Jaundice
Check bilirubin on blood sample if:
- Jaundice at < 24 hours of age
- Looks significantly jaundiced clinically
- Significant level on transcutaneous monitor

Septic spots
White spots – erythema toxicum or milia are common and harmless
Septic spots – contain pus
Bullous impetigo – serious (staphylococcal or streptococcal) infection. Sacs of serous fluid; their roof is easily broken leaving denuded skin

Pallor/plethora
- Check hematocrit for anemia or polycythemia
- Check breathing and circulation

Jitteriness/seizures/lethargy
Jittery movements are common – if pronounced check blood glucose and consider other causes, e.g. drug withdrawal
Seizures can be subtle, but are rhythmic jerky movements of the limbs which cannot be stopped on holding
Requires prompt treatment and investigation – admit to the neonatal unit
Lethargy may be a sign of sepsis, hypoglycemia or inborn error of metabolism

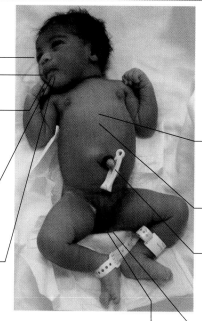

Delay in passing meconium (> 24 hours)
Check for intestinal obstruction

Delay in voiding urine (> 24 hours)
Voiding may be unobserved – often void immediately after birth
Consider urinary outflow obstruction (palpable bladder, ultrasound) or renal failure (serum creatinine, ultrasound)

Weight loss
Babies initially lose weight (1–2% of birth weight per day up to 7–10% of birth weight). They take 10–14 days to regain their birth weight

Collapse (rare but important)
Maintain Airway, Breathing, Circulation
Causes:
- Sepsis – bacterial or viral
- Duct-dependent heart disease – closure of ductus arteriosus
- Inborn error of metabolism

Hypoglycemia
Blood glucose < 40 mg/dL (< 2.6 mmol/L) and asymptomatic – feed infant and recheck
If symptomatic, blood glucose levels are very low < 20 mg/dL (1.1 mmol/L) or persistently < 40 mg/dL (< 2.6 mmol/L) despite adequate feeding – give intravenous glucose

Respiratory distress
Most common cause – TTNB (transient tachypnea of the newborn), but need to exclude infection and other causes
Check Airway, Breathing, Circulation
Give oxygen, respiratory and circulatory support as required
Admit to neonatal unit
Check – complete blood count, blood culture, C-reactive protein and chest X-ray
Start antibiotics

Apneic attacks
The pauses in normal periodic breathing are sometimes misinterpreted as apnea by parents
True apnea with desaturation is uncommon in term infants and is a serious symptom; infection must be excluded

Umbilical cord
Red flare in skin around umbilicus – usually staphylococcal or streptococcal. Give intravenous antibiotics

The septic baby
A combination of some of these clinical features:
- Apnea and bradycardia
- Slow feeding or vomiting or abdominal distension
- Fever, hypothermia or temperature instability
- Respiratory distress
- Irritability, lethargy or seizures
- Jaundice
- Petechiae or bruising
- Reduced limb movement (bone or joint infection)
- Collapse or shock
- Hypoglycemia
In meningitis (late signs):
- Tense or bulging fontanelle
- Head retraction (opisthotonus)
Admit to neonatal unit
Check – complete blood count, blood and other cultures, C-reactive protein and chest X-ray
Consider lumbar puncture
Start antibiotics
Provide supportive therapy

Fig. 21.1 Common medical problems of term infants.

Newborn infants should not be separated from their mothers unless it is essential for their well-being. Additional nursing and medical care can be provided on postpartum (postnatal) wards or by providing transitional care facilities beside their mother. However, 6–10% of newborn infants are admitted to a neonatal unit and 1–2% require intensive care.

Families often find neonatal units daunting and frightening. The environment is unfamiliar and their small and fragile baby is surrounded by high-tech equipment. There are large numbers of highly skilled nurses, doctors and other health professionals caring for their baby, and parents and families often feel superfluous as they are unable to help and care for their baby. Much can be done for parents and families to avoid these difficulties or help them cope with them.

Welcoming parents and families

• Parents and families should always be made welcome by staff (however busy they are).

Open access

• Open visiting policy for parents (Fig. 22.1) and ability to exchange information 24 hours per day. Mothers should be transported to be near their baby.
• Visits by grandparents (Fig. 22.2) and close family members as well as supervised sibling visits (Fig. 22.3) should be encouraged.

Explanation and facilitating communication

• Explain the infant's medical condition and equipment. Provide written information.
• Check with parents how they think their baby is doing and determine their level of understanding about their infant's condition and care. Correct misconceptions. Listen to the parents. Use interpreters if necessary.
• Arrange privacy for more detailed discussions. Parents appreciate respect for personal values and being involved in decision-making as appropriate.
• Assist the family to experience their new baby as a person by

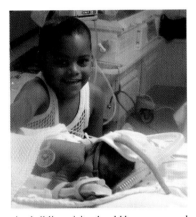
Fig. 22.2 Grandparents on the neonatal unit visiting the latest additions to their family.

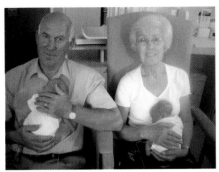
Fig. 22.3 Supervised sibling visits should be encouraged.

visualizing the infant beyond the tubes and devices.
• Utilize other professionals, e.g. counselors, social workers. They may also provide helpful liaison between the neonatal intensive care unit (NICU) team and family as they may be perceived by the family as being less threatening than health-care professionals.
• The primary nurse, who is responsible for that baby, facilitates identification of areas of concern and organizes discharge.
• Arrange care conferences with the family, including all subspecialists involved in the care of infants with complex problems. These meetings are invaluable in keeping the family up to date and planning for discharge and subsequent care.

Assisting attachment

• Give the mother the opportunity to touch and hold her baby in delivery room, if at all possible.
• Encourage the mother to express breast milk. This enables her to participate directly in her baby's care. Success depends on support and encouragement by staff.
• Promote touching of infant (Fig. 22.4), even on ventilator (Fig. 22.5).
• Encourage parents to actively participate in their infant's care (Fig. 22.6). When the baby is stable enough, parents may hold their baby during feeding (Fig. 22.7) and provide kangaroo care (Fig. 22.8a and

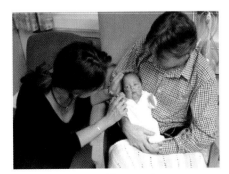
Fig. 22.1 Encourage parents to visit at any time.

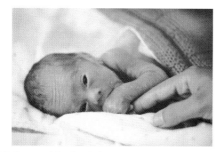

Fig. 22.4 Mother touching her infant.

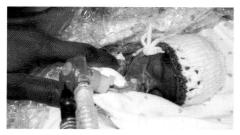

Fig. 22.5 Mother touching her ventilated infant.

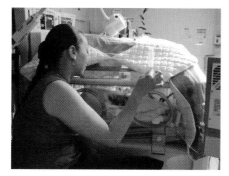

Fig. 22.6 Mother gavage (tube) feeding her ill baby.

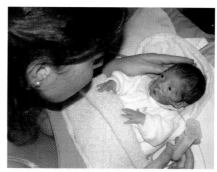

Fig. 22.7 Mother gavage (tube) feeding her baby.

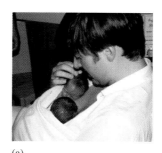 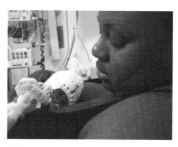

(a)   (b)

Fig. 22.8 (a and b) Kangaroo care, with direct skin-to-skin contact with parent. In some developing countries where isolettes (incubators) are not available, prolonged use has been shown to reduce mortality.

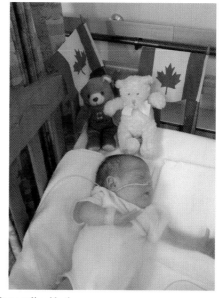

Fig. 22.9 Personalized bed.

b). Individualized nursing plans address the baby's behavioral and environmental needs and may reduce morbidity and length of stay (see Chapter 23).

• Leave notes for parents from their baby (with parental agreement). Refer to the baby by name. Ensure the family is provided with good quality photos of their baby. Personalize the isolette (incubator) with family pictures, religious texts etc. (Fig. 22.9). Offer to keep diary of baby's milestone events.

Providing a family-friendly environment

• Make appearance of the unit as family-friendly as possible.
• Provide space and facilities for parents and families to have some privacy with their baby.
• Try to simulate a nurturing environment, as in one's home – avoid noise in the unit, avoid sunlight on babies, make the unit darker at night.

• Provide facilities for families to relax near but separate from the unit, with play area for siblings.
• Provide rooms for parents to stay overnight. This is particularly important if their infant is critically ill or prior to discharge.

Developmental care complements high-tech medical and nursing care. It involves tailoring care to fit the infant's needs and abilities rather than the convenience of caregivers or institutions. The aim is to improve the infant's developmental potential by enhancing the physical and social environment. It is multidisciplinary and embodies a family-centered and child-centered approach.

Brain development

In the newborn, particularly if preterm, the brain is developing rapidly and is at a peak period of forming new neuronal connections. This process depends partly on experience. Individualized developmental care aims to provide experience appropriate for the infant's stage of neurodevelopment and to optimize neurodevelopmental potential.

The family

The early relationship (attachment) between infant and parents is important for healthy emotional and social development. Developmental care can help parents to understand their baby's needs and to become confident through facilitated interaction with their baby. There are many different styles of parenting, and many different ways in which parents cope with the trauma of having a baby in special or intensive care. Respecting these differences and needs is part of family-centered care.

Observing newborn behavior

Developmental readiness for experience can be gauged by observing the baby's behavior and the context in which it occurs. Sensitivity to the infant's behavioral cues is the foundation of developmental care. Changes in physiologic balance, motor activity, states of arousal and attentiveness suggest the infant's ability to cope with a situation. The baby may show behaviors that appear to be signs of readiness to interact and competence in self-regulating (approach behavior) or to be defensive or withdrawing (avoidance behavior) (Table 23.1).

The nursery environment

The premature infant is not suited to bright light, loud noise, hard surfaces, and the many sudden stimuli typical of neonatal intensive care units. These experiences can be modified, e.g. lighting can be subdued and isolettes (incubators) covered (Fig. 23.2), noise can be reduced with sound-absorbing materials and staff can be encouraged to talk and work quietly. Nesting with soft bedding can provide comforting boundaries (Fig. 23.3).

Table 23.1 Behavioral observation.

	Approach behavior	**Avoidance behavior**
Autonomic	Regular, gentle breathing	Breathing irregular, fast, labored
	Healthy pink coloring	Pale, dusky, flushed or mottled
	Comfortable digestion	Straining, gagging, vomiting
Motor	Smooth varied movement	Jerky, disorganized movement
	Softly flexed posture	Extended (Fig. 23.1b) or flat posture
	Modulated muscle tone	Flaccid or stiff tone
State	Restful sleep	Diffuse, disorganized state
	Periodic sleep/wake pattern	Restless sleep
	Quiet alertness	Frequent state changes
Attention	Sustained, focussed alertness (Fig. 23.1a)	Glazed, strained, hyperalert look
Self-regulation	Self-calming	Inconsolable
	Socially responsive	Shut down

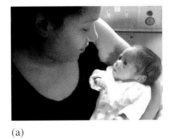
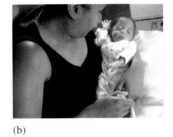

(a)   (b)

Fig. 23.1 (a) This baby's controlled posture and focussed expression show successful self-regulation and readiness for interaction, i.e. approach behavior. (b) Extended limbs and turning away suggest avoidance behavior.

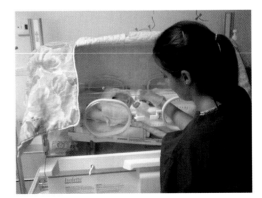

Fig. 23.2 Isolette (incubator) covered to provide subdued lighting. A flap is raised so that the baby can be observed.

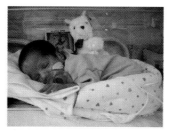

Fig. 23.3 Soft bedding with supportive nesting can contain disorganized movement and provide the baby with comforting boundaries.

Adapting care

Care can be adjusted to fit the baby's abilities and sensitivity (Fig. 23.4). Infants in intensive care are frequently disturbed for nursing observations, examinations, diaper (nappy) changes, blood and other tests, giving medications, etc. Procedures can often be performed together to minimize disturbing the baby, even if this means being flexible about timing routine observations and cares, or performing tests and therapy. Timing and pacing of procedures can be adjusted according to the behavioral cues that show when the baby needs time out to rest and recover from difficult procedures. Infants can also be helped to cope with unpleasant or painful experiences by providing comforting boundaries, opportunities to suck and a calm environment (see Chapter 61). Sensitive infants may initially be helped to find bathing pleasurable if contained (Fig. 23.5).

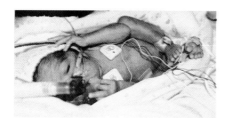

Fig. 23.4 Many activities can be done with the baby lying on one side to give more control of movement.

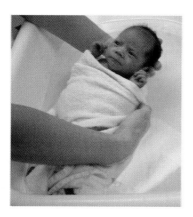

Fig. 23.5 Help sensitive infants to find bathing pleasurable by containing them within a loosely wrapped towel.

Parent participation

Parents are the baby's most consistent and dedicated carers. As they begin to recognize their baby's individual characteristics, strengths and sensitivities, they can be encouraged to provide care that is appropriate for the baby's state and level of development. Even if the infant is receiving intensive care, they can usually become involved with their baby's care at the earliest stage, for example by comforting the baby with still hands, or by helping with mouth care or giving a gavage (tube) feed. As soon as the infant is sufficiently stable, parents should be offered the opportunity to cuddle their baby. Parental involvement in the provision of care increases as their baby becomes more stable and mature (Figs 23.6 and 23.7).

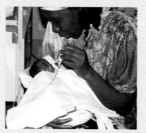 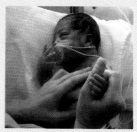

Fig. 23.6 Promotion of parental attachment by involvement with their baby's care.

Fig. 23.7 Promotion of parental attachment through touch and massage.

Questions

What is the Newborn Behavioral Assessment Scale (NBAS)?
It includes a variety of tasks that demonstrate infant maturity and individuality. Habituation, orientation to visual and auditory stimuli, motor maturity and reflex responses are tested and the baby's responses to increasingly challenging situations are noted. The examiner must be skillful in eliciting the baby's best response as well as in scoring the assessment.

What is NIDCAP®?
This is the Newborn Individualized Developmental Care and Assessment Program developed by Dr Heidelise Als and colleagues. NIDCAP® practitioners have formal training in systematic observation and treatment planning, leading to a certificate of reliability. NIDCAP® emphasizes individualized care. A number of studies in the US, Canada and Sweden have shown improved outcomes.

Seriously ill or extremely preterm infants may require resuscitation. Thereafter, they all need to be promptly stabilized and therapy should be initiated for organ-specific dysfunction (Fig. 24.1).

Airway, Breathing
Examination
▪ Respiratory distress – respiratory rate, chest retractions, nasal flaring, grunting
Treatment as required with:
▫ Clearing the airway
▫ Oxygen
▫ CPAP
▫ Mechanical ventilation

Give surfactant therapy as indicated

Circulation
Examination
▪ Heart rate, pulses, capillary refill time, skin color and temperature
▪ Blood pressure
Treat shock – see facing page

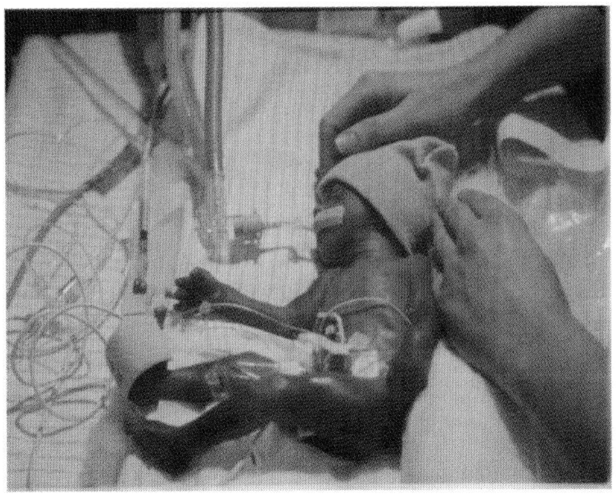

Venous and arterial lines
Peripheral intravenous line
▪ Required for intravenous fluids, antibiotics, other drugs and parenteral nutrition
Umbilical venous catheter
▪ Sometimes used for immediate intravenous access or for CVP (central venous pressure) monitoring or obtaining blood samples or administration of fluid or medications. Some centers use multilumen catheters to avoid the need for peripheral IV lines, but they carry a higher risk of infection and thrombosis than peripheral lines
Arterial line
▪ Inserted if frequent blood gas analysis, blood tests and continuous blood pressure monitoring is required. Usually umbilical artery catheter (UAC), sometimes peripheral cannula if for short period or no umbilical artery catheter possible. Continuous arterial blood gas monitoring has been developed
Central venous line for parenteral nutrition
▪ Inserted peripherally when infant is stable

Central nervous system
Examination
▪ Response to handling
▫ Posture
▪ Movements
▫ Tone
▪ Reflexes

X-rays
Chest X-ray ± abdominal X-ray assist in cause of respiratory distress, position of tracheal tube and central lines

Monitoring
▫ Oxygen saturation
▪ Heart rate
▪ Respiratory rate
▫ Temperature
▪ Blood pressure
▪ Blood glucose
▪ Blood gases
▪ Weight
▪ Transcutaneous O_2 and CO_2 – used in some centers

Antibiotics
Usually given before results of cultures and other investigations are available (although most infants are not septic)

Pain/sedation
Analgesia and sedation given according to assessment of need, e.g. painful procedures, artificial ventilation
Muscle relaxants may sometimes be required during mechanical ventilation

Temperature control
To keep the infant warm, stabilization is performed under a radiant warmer or in an isolette (incubator)

Parents
Time needs to be found to explain to parents and immediate relatives what is happening. If the mother cannot see the baby, e.g. following cesarean section or severe hypertension, photographs or videolinks are reassuring

Investigations
▪ Hemoglobin/Hematocrit
▪ Neutrophil count
▪ Platelets
▪ Blood urea nitrogen (BUN)/creatinine
▪ Electrolytes
▪ Culture – blood ± CSF ± urine
▪ Blood glucose
▪ CRP/acute phase reactant
▪ Surface cultures
▪ Coagulation screen if indicated

Vitamin K
Routine prophylaxis against hemorrhagic disease of the newborn

Fig. 24.1 Stabilizing the newborn infant requiring intensive care.

Oxygen saturation

What arterial oxygen saturation should one aim for?

This depends on the infant's maturity and underlying clinical condition.
- Healthy term infants have an oxygen saturation >97%.
- Term infants with cyanotic congenital heart disease tolerate saturations of around 80%.
- Preterm infants – oxygen saturation between 88 and 95% is compatible with adequate oxygen tension and this range is widely adopted.
- Preterm infants receiving supplemental oxygen must be monitored with arterial oxygen tension measurements to detect hypoxemia and because high saturations may represent high tissue oxygen tensions (Fig. 24.2), which are potentially dangerous to the eyes (retinopathy of prematurity) and lungs (bronchopulmonary dysplasia, chronic lung disease).

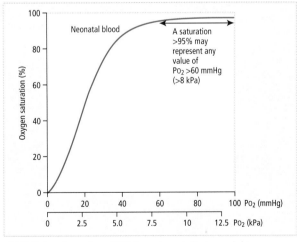

Neonatal blood

A saturation >95% may represent any value of P_{O_2} >60 mmHg (>8 kPa)

Fig. 24.2 Saturations above 95% in preterm infants receiving supplemental oxygen may represent dangerously high oxygen tensions.

Heart rate

What information can be obtained by monitoring heart rate? (Table 24.1)

Interpreting the heart rate is best done in conjunction with respiratory rate and oxygen saturation. Episodes of desaturation are mostly transient or from movement artifact, but if more severe and prolonged will be accompanied by bradycardia and require prompt attention.

Circulation

How is the need for circulatory support determined?

The causes of shock are shown in Fig. 24.3. The clinical signs of shock are difficult to interpret.

The circulation is assessed by:

- Heart rate – usually tachycardia in shock; bradycardia is a late sign.
- Temperature gap: central – peripheral i.e. tummy–toe, difference >2°C. Also caused by a cold environment. Capillary refill time is prolonged if >3 seconds in neonates.
- Blood pressure measurement – hypotension. But central blood pressure correlates poorly with circulating blood volume.
- Metabolic acidosis (increased lactate levels).
- Oliguria.
- Echocardiography – used increasingly to help identify underfilling suggesting hypovolemia and/or poor contractility from myocardial dysfunction.
- Chest X-ray – excludes pneumothorax, diaphragmatic hernia.

Cardiovascular function may be compromised by overinflation of lungs or high mean airway pressure on mechanical ventilation obstructing venous return.

A management regimen is shown in Fig. 24.4.

Table 24.1 Some causes of isolated changes in heart rate.

Increased heart rate (>160 beats/minute)
Movement/crying
Respiratory distress
Hypovolemia
Fever, infection
Pain
Fluid overload, e.g. heart failure, patent ductus arteriosus
Supraventricular tachycardia
Anemia
Thyrotoxicosis

Decreased heart rate (<100 beats/minute)
Apnea, hypoxia
Seizures
Shock (uncompensated)
Heart block, arrhythmia
Raised intracranial pressure
Hypothermia
Artefact

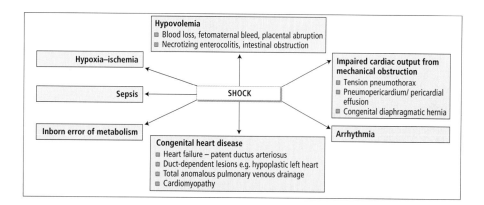

Fig. 24.3 Causes of shock.

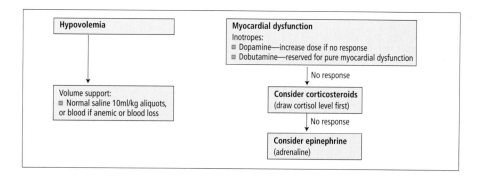

Fig. 24.4 Example of management regimen for circulatory support.

Forms of respiratory support

These are:
- Supplemental oxygen
- CPAP – continuous positive airway pressure
- Positive pressure ventilation
- HFOV – high-frequency oscillatory ventilation
- NO – nitric oxide
- ECMO – extracorporeal membrane oxygenation.

Although many new forms of respiratory support are becoming available, teams of professionals fully familiar with a limited range of equipment are likely to have better outcomes than those using an array of sophisticated new equipment with which they are not fully conversant.

The increase in use of nasal CPAP and HFOV as respiratory support for very low birthweight (VLBW) infants is shown in Fig. 25.1. It also shows the change in use of other respiratory interventions; the increased use of surfactant (see Chapter 27) and recent decline in use of postnatal corticosteroids (see Chapter 36).

Supplemental oxygen therapy

- Oxygen is given to treat hypoxemia (Figs 25.2 and 25.3), with the goal of avoiding arterial oxygen tension (PaO_2) of <45 mmHg

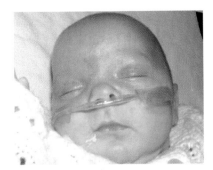

Fig. 25.3 Nasal cannula to deliver oxygen.

(6 kPa) or arterial oxygen saturation (SpO_2) of <88%.
- Term infants are maintained at oxygen saturation >97%.
- In preterm infants, maintaining the arterial oxygen tension at 45–80 mmHg (6.0–10.5 kPa) and saturation 88–95% is usually recommended.

Continuous positive airway pressure (CPAP)

Distending pressure is usually applied via either nasal prongs (Fig. 25.4) or a tracheal tube in the nasal airway. CPAP aims to prevent alveolar collapse at end expiration. It also allows supplemental oxygen to be delivered continuously. It is used for infants with moder-

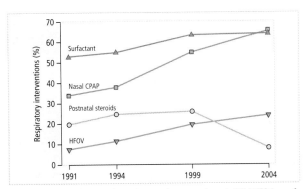

Fig. 25.1 Changes in use of respiratory interventions in VLBW (very low birthweight) infants with time. (Vermont–Oxford Network; courtesy of Dr Jeff Horbar.)

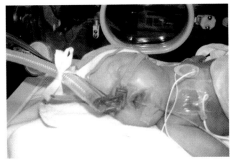

Fig. 25.4 Nasal CPAP (continuous positive airway pressure). Some circuits have a fluidic flip, whereby the direction of air flow reverses during expiration. This reduces the work of breathing. Another system is bubble CPAP, in which the pressure is regulated using an underwater manometer.

Table 25.1 Some practical details about CPAP.

Start with 5–6 cm H_2O pressure and increase as necessary
Pass nasogastric or orogastric tube – leave on free drainage to reduce gaseous distension of the stomach
Weaning from CPAP – first reduce oxygen concentration, then airway pressure

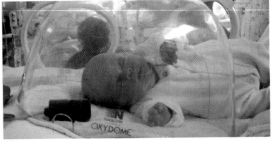

Fig. 25.2 Oxygen via hood. Advantage – simple to administer. Disadvantages – confining, hot, not possible to maintain high oxygen concentration.

ate respiratory distress and for recurrent apnea (Table 25.1). It may allow weaning from mechanical ventilation.

Complications of CPAP are:
- pneumothorax
- feeding difficulties due to gaseous distention of the stomach
- often poorly tolerated by term infants.

If respiratory failure develops, mechanical ventilation is required.

Some infants with bronchopulmonary dysplasia (chronic lung disease) require nasal CPAP for many weeks. Prolonged use of nasal prongs may cause nasal trauma, long-term damage to the nasal septum and deformity of the nose. Correct fixation will minimize this.

Even with extremely preterm infants, there is a trend to starting nasal CPAP immediately after birth and intubating only if necessary.

Positive pressure ventilation

Intermittent positive pressure ventilation (IPPV)

Ventilatory support is administered using a mechanical ventilator through a tracheal tube. Intermittent positive pressure ventilator breaths are given on a background of continuous distending pressure (positive end expiratory pressure, PEEP) (Fig. 25.5). Alveolar ventilation is determined by the difference between peak inspiratory pressure (PIP) and PEEP, the inspiratory time and respiratory rate.

Most neonatal ventilators are pressure-limited and time-cycled. They are used as tracheal tubes are not cuffed and so there is an air leak.

Volume-limited ventilators can be used in neonates and are used in some neonatal units.

Patient-triggered (assist/control) ventilation and synchronous intermittent mandatory ventilation

Two forms of synchronized mechanical ventilation are available to promote synchrony between the ventilator and a baby's own respi-

ratory efforts – patient-triggered ventilation (PTV) and synchronous intermittent mandatory ventilation (SIMV). Both methods use a baby's own spontaneous respiration to trigger the ventilator to deliver a breath, usually from the change in airway pressure or flow measured in the ventilator circuit; or from a recording of the infant's respiration. In PTV each breath triggers the ventilator; in SIMV only a preset number of breaths in a given time are triggered. In both, there is a backup ventilation rate if the infant does not breathe.

Multicenter studies have failed to show any advantages of PTV or SIMV over conventional ventilation for preterm infants with respiratory distress syndrome, although these forms of ventilation may decrease the need for sedation.

High-frequency oscillatory ventilation (HFOV)

High-frequency ventilators operate at frequencies approximately 10 times greater than conventional ventilators and can achieve good gas exchange despite using tidal volumes smaller than dead space (Fig 25.6). The rationale for using high-frequency ventilation is to recruit collapsed alveoli and minimize ventilator-induced lung damage. Rescue treatment with high-frequency ventilation in term and preterm infants with severe respiratory failure is associated with short-term improvement in gas exchange, especially when used in combination with inhaled nitric oxide. Some units choose to ventilate all their extremely preterm infants by HFOV to minimize barotrauma. Studies have failed to show a decrease in duration of ventilation, incidence of bronchopulmonary dysplasia (chronic lung disease), mortality or need for extracorporeal membrane oxygenation (ECMO) compared with conventional ventilation.

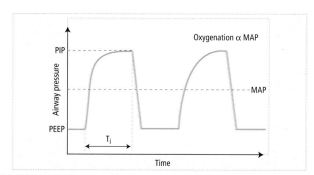

Fig. 25.5 Intermittent positive pressure ventilation (IPPV). Diagram of change in airway pressure with time. (PIP – peak inspiratory pressure; PEEP – positive end-expiratory pressure; Ti – inspiratory time; MAP – mean airway pressure.)

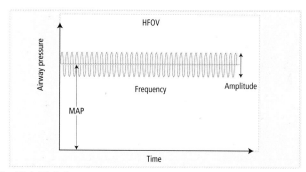

Fig. 25.6 High-frequency oscillatory ventilation (HFOV). Diagram showing changes in airway pressure with time. (MAP – mean airway pressure.)

Mechanical ventilation – indications and complications

Indications

- Increasing oxygen requirement or work of breathing or increasing $PaCO_2$ while on nasal CPAP.
- Respiratory failure – defect in oxygenation (hypoxemia) and/or carbon dioxide elimination (hypercarbia).
- Apnea – prolonged/recurrent.
- Upper airway obstruction.
- Congenital diaphragmatic hernia.
- Circulatory failure.

Causes of sudden deterioration

- Tracheal tube blocked/displaced.
- Ventilator/circuit disconnected or malfunction.
- Air leak – tension pneumothorax (Fig. 25.7) or pneumo-mediastinum.
- Pulmonary hemorrhage.
- Hemorrhage – intraventricular or other sites.

Causes of slow deterioration

- Increased lung secretions.
- Infection.
- Patent ductus arteriosus.
- Anemia.
- Developing bronchopulmonary dysplasia (chronic lung disease).

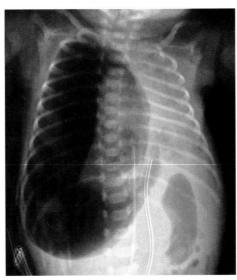

Fig. 25.7 Chest X-ray showing large right-sided tension pneumothorax. The mediastinum and umbilical venous and arterial lines are displaced to the left.

Minimizing ventilator- and oxygen-induced lung injury

Minimize ventilator-induced lung injury (exudates, inflammation, air leaks) by:
- avoiding inappropriately high inflation pressures by:
  - use of low inflation pressures and tolerating higher arterial pCO_2 values – but too low pressures can also be damaging, from ventilating atelectatic lung
  - high-frequency oscillatory ventilation

  However, neither technique has been shown to be superior in reducing bronchopulmonary dysplasia (chronic lung disease).
- trying to synchronize the ventilator with the infant's breathing – by trying to match their rates, or with synchronized ventilation. Analgesics, e.g. morphine or sedatives, may be given to decrease pain, agitation or spontaneous respiratory effort. For very severe lung disease or restlessness in mature infants, muscle relaxants are sometimes given as well, but are generally avoided as they result in marked peripheral edema.

Avoid oxygen-induced lung damage from free radical injury by using the minimum concentration of oxygen necessary. Preterm infants are particularly vulnerable as they have inadequate antioxidant defense mechanisms.

Respiratory failure

The severity of hypoxemic respiratory failure is assessed by calculating the oxygenation index (OI):

$$OI = \frac{\text{mean airway pressure (cm } H_2O) \times FiO_2 \times 100}{PaO_2 \text{ (mmHg)}}$$

In term infants OI ≥40 is associated with a 40% risk of mortality.
In preterm infants OI ≥20 is associated with a 50% risk of mortality.

Therapeutic options for respiratory failure if on conventional mechanical ventilation with high pressures and high concentration of oxygen are:
- extra rescue doses of surfactant
- high-frequency ventilation
- nitric oxide therapy
- ECMO for infants of ≥35 weeks' gestation.

Inhaled nitric oxide (iNO)

Nitric oxide is an endogenous vasodilator. It is used in infants with hypoxemic respiratory failure with or without persistent pulmonary hypertension of the newborn (PPHN) to improve oxygenation (Fig. 25.8). Inhaled NO (iNO) reduces the need for ECMO in term and near-term infants with severe respiratory failure. Its efficacy in preterm infants is controversial.

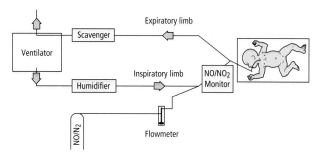

Fig. 25.8 Circuit for delivering nitric oxide. There is a scavenger for removing nitric oxide released into the atmosphere. The blood concentration of methemoglobin, a potentially toxic byproduct, is checked periodically. Inspired nitrogen dioxide (NO_2) levels (a byproduct of mixing nitric oxide and oxygen) are monitored continuously.

Question

What is nitric oxide (NO) and why is it useful?

It is produced endogenously by vascular endothelium and causes vascular smooth muscle relaxation.

Inhaled nitric oxide causes selective pulmonary vasodilation.

It lowers pulmonary vascular resistance and improves arterial oxygenation.

Extracorporeal membrane oxygenation (ECMO)

Infants are placed on heart–lung bypass for up to several days to allow the lungs to recover (Fig. 25.9). It is performed in relatively few specialized centers. Because of the need for anticoagulation, there is a risk of intraventricular hemorrhage in preterm infants and it is therefore reserved for infants ≥35 weeks' gestation and birth weight >2 kg. Indication is an oxygenation index of ≥30–40. Conditions that may result in respiratory failure and need ECMO are listed in Table 25.2. The need for ECMO has declined markedly since the introduction of nitric oxide and HFOV and the reduced incidence of severe meconium aspiration syndrome.

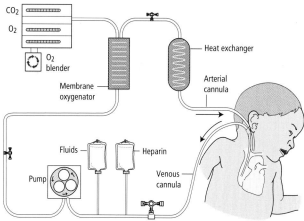

Fig. 25.9 ECMO (extracorporeal membrane oxygenation) circuit. The infant's venous blood is drained by gravity and pumped through a membrane oxygenator (an artificial lung), which extracts carbon dioxide and adds oxygen. The blood is returned to the baby through an artery (venoarterial ECMO, as shown in the diagram) or a vein (venovenous ECMO). The lungs continue to be ventilated but at a low resting level. The carotid artery is often ligated for venoarterial ECMO, which carries a risk of ischemic brain injury.

Table 25.2 Conditions that may require ECMO.

Severe respiratory failure from:
- meconium aspiration syndrome
- persistent pulmonary hypertension of the newborn (PPHN)
- sepsis
- respiratory distress syndrome (RDS)
- congenital diaphragmatic hernia
- heart disease – congenital or cardiomyopathy
- severe airway obstruction/malformation

Key point

Only one randomized controlled trial on ECMO (UK ECMO Trial), which showed that it reduced mortality from 59 to 32% without increasing long-term disability.

26 The preterm infant

The preterm infant differs markedly from the term infant in size, appearance and development. Some of these differences are shown schematically in Figs 26.1–4.

Gestation	23–25 weeks	29–31 weeks	37–42 weeks (term)
Birthweight (50th centile)	At 24 weeks – Female: 620 g; Male: 700 g	At 30 weeks – Female: 1.4 kg; Male: 1.5 kg	At 40 weeks – Female: 3.4 kg; Male: 3.55 kg
Skin	Very thin, gelatinous. Dark red all over body	Medium thickness Pink	Thick skin with cracking on hands and feet. Pale pink: pink all over ears, lips, palms and soles
Ears	Pinna soft, no recoil	Cartilage to edge of pinna in places, recoils readily	Firm pinna cartilage to edge of pinna, recoils immediately
Breast	No breast tissue palpable	One or both breast nodules 0.5–1.0 cm	One or both nodules > 1.0 cm
Genitalia	Male: scrotum smooth, testes impalpable. Female: prominent clitoris. Labia majora widely separated, labia minora protruding	Male: scrotum – few rugae, testes – inguinal canal. Female: labia minora and clitoris partially covered	Male: scrotum – rugae, testes in scrotum. Female: labia minora and clitoris covered
Posture	Extended, jerky, uncoordinated	Some flexion of legs	Flexed, smooth limb movements
Vision	Eyelids may be fused or partially open. Absent or infrequent eye movements	Pupils react to light	Looks at faces. Follows faces, curvy lines and light/dark contrast in all directions
Hearing	Startles to loud noise		Turns head and eyes to sound. Prefers speech and mother's voice
Breathing	Needs respiratory support. Apnea common	Sometimes needs respiratory support. Apnea common	Need for respiratory support uncommon. Apnea rare
Sucking and swallowing	No coordinated sucking		Coordinated at 34–35 weeks' gestation
Feeding	Usually need TPN (total parenteral nutrition)	Gavage (nasogastric) feeds. Sometimes need TPN (total parenteral nutrition)	At term, cries when hungry. Takes full feeds on demand. Coordinates breathing, sucking and swallowing
Taste		Reacts to bitter taste	Differentiates between sweet, sour, bitter. Prefers sweet
Interaction	Seldom available for interaction. Easily overloaded by sensory stimulation		Makes eye contact and alert wakefulness
Cry	Very faint		Loud
Sleep/wake cycle	Intermediate sleep state		Clearly defined sleeping and waking states

Fig. 26.1 Maturational changes in appearance and development with age.

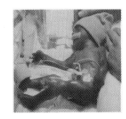

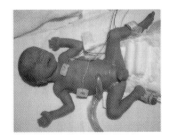

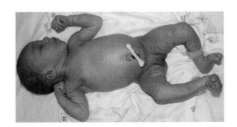

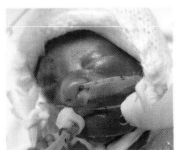

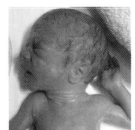

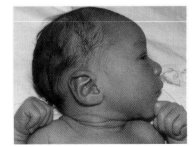

Fig. 26.2 Preterm infant at 23 weeks' gestation, showing extended posture, thin, gelatinous skin and fused eyelids.

Fig. 26.3 Preterm infant at 30 weeks' gestation, showing medium-thickness skin and ear with cartilage to edge of pinna.

Fig. 26.4 Term infant showing flexed posture and thick skin, and well-formed ear.

Morbidity

Being born preterm has many disadvantages, including stress for the parents and family, prolonged hospitalization and considerable expense. After 30 weeks of gestation, most preterm infants in developed countries survive without neurologic impairment. However, at lower gestational age there is considerable morbidity (Fig. 26.5). The morbidity is highly dependent on gestational age (Fig. 26.6).

Mortality

Mortality is mainly determined by gestational age (see Figs. 2.3a and 37.1) and birth weight (Fig. 26.7). They interact with each other as well as with other risk factors:

- gender (males have higher mortality)
- ethnicity
- multiple birth.

There has been a marked improvement in survival in infants born at the limit of viability, i.e. 23–25 weeks of gestational age, birth weight 500–800 grams. However, mortality, morbidity and adverse neurodevelopmental outcome are highest in these infants. This is considered further in Chapters 2 and 69.

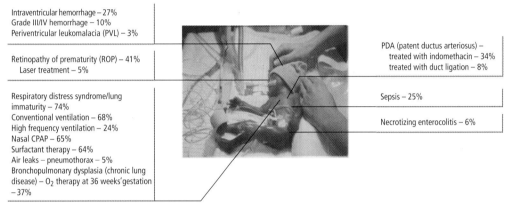

Intraventricular hemorrhage – 27%
Grade III/IV hemorrhage – 10%
Periventricular leukomalacia (PVL) – 3%

Retinopathy of prematurity (ROP) – 41%
Laser treatment – 5%

Respiratory distress syndrome/lung immaturity – 74%
Conventional ventilation – 68%
High frequency ventilation – 24%
Nasal CPAP – 65%
Surfactant therapy – 64%
Air leaks – pneumothorax – 5%
Bronchopulmonary dysplasia (chronic lung disease) – O_2 therapy at 36 weeks' gestation – 37%

PDA (patent ductus arteriosus) – treated with indomethacin – 34% treated with duct ligation – 8%

Sepsis – 25%

Necrotizing enterocolitis – 6%

Fig. 26.5 Complications in the neonatal unit in very low birthweight (<1.5 kg) infants. (Percentages are based on Vermont–Oxford Network data, 2004.)

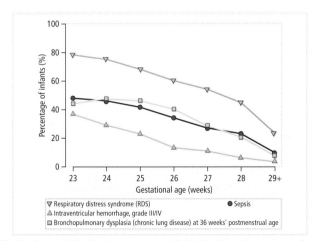

Fig. 26.6 Morbidity in the neonatal unit is highly dependent on gestational age. (NICHD Neonatal Research Network 1997–2000.)

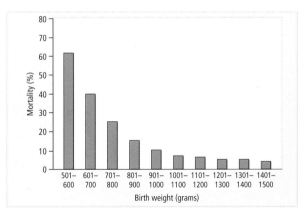

Fig. 26.7 Mortality by birthweight in very low birthweight (VLBW) infants. (Vermont–Oxford Network, 2004.)

27 Lung development and surfactant

Structural development

The fetal lung passes through four main stages of lung development during gestation (Fig. 27.1).

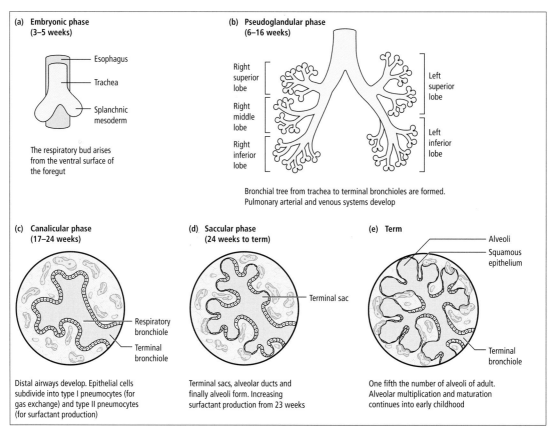

(a) Embryonic phase (3–5 weeks)

Esophagus
Trachea
Splanchnic mesoderm

The respiratory bud arises from the ventral surface of the foregut

(b) Pseudoglandular phase (6–16 weeks)

Right superior lobe
Right middle lobe
Right inferior lobe
Left superior lobe
Left inferior lobe

Bronchial tree from trachea to terminal bronchioles are formed. Pulmonary arterial and venous systems develop

(c) Canalicular phase (17–24 weeks)

Respiratory bronchiole
Terminal bronchiole

Distal airways develop. Epithelial cells subdivide into type I pneumocytes (for gas exchange) and type II pneumocytes (for surfactant production)

(d) Saccular phase (24 weeks to term)

Terminal sac

Terminal sacs, alveolar ducts and finally alveoli form. Increasing surfactant production from 23 weeks

(e) Term

Alveoli
Squamous epithelium
Terminal bronchiole

One fifth the number of alveoli of adult. Alveolar multiplication and maturation continues into early childhood

Fig. 27.1 Phases of lung development.

Physiology and composition of surfactant (Figs 27.2–4)

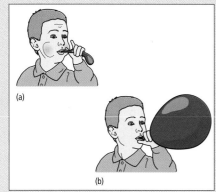

(a)

(b)

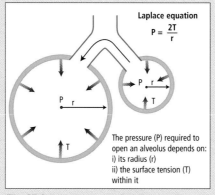

Laplace equation

$$P = \frac{2T}{r}$$

The pressure (P) required to open an alveolus depends on:
i) its radius (r)
ii) the surface tension (T) within it

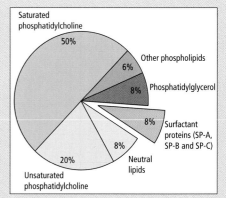

Saturated phosphatidylcholine 50%
Other phospholipids 6%
Phosphatidylglycerol 8%
Surfactant proteins (SP-A, SP-B and SP-C) 8%
Neutral lipids 8%
Unsaturated phosphatidylcholine 20%

Fig. 27.2 (a) It is hard to blow up a balloon that is collapsed, i.e. has a small radius. Surfactant-deficient lungs are like this. (b) It is easier to blow up once the balloon is partially filled with air, i.e. has a larger radius. Lungs with surfactant are like this.

Fig. 27.3 In the absence of surfactant, the pressure at the surface of the alveolus is greater in the smaller than the larger alveolus, so the small alveoli collapse and the large ones expand. Surfactant lowers the surface tension (T) and prevents alveolar collapse.

Fig. 27.4 Composition of surfactant.

Surfactant

Surfactant:

• is a naturally occurring substance containing lipids (90%) and proteins (10%)

• is synthesized in type II pneumocytes in the lung and released onto the alveolar surface

• lowers surface tension at the air–water interface in the alveolus through the action of its lipid components (mainly dipalmitoyl phosphatidylcholine, DPPC). This effect helps to prevent alveolar collapse (atelectasis) and improves lung compliance (lung stiffness), reducing the work of breathing

• is only produced late in the second trimester and early third trimester

• deficiency causes respiratory distress syndrome (RDS).

Clinical implications of surfactant deficiency

In surfactant deficiency, as the lung has low compliance (i.e. it is stiff), the change in lung volume for a given change in airway pressure is much less than in the normal healthy newborn lung (Fig. 27.5). The pressure required to initiate lung inflation ('opening pressure') is also higher. Without surfactant the lung alveoli collapse to zero volume during expiration and the next breath starts from a low lung volume. These changes result in increased work of breathing and hypoxemia (Fig 27.6).

Antenatal corticosteroids

Promote surfactant synthesis and lung maturation. They reduce the incidence of RDS by 60% and mortality by 40%. There is no increase in infection rate or maternal adverse side effects. The maximum benefit is when given more than 24 hours before delivery. It is uncertain whether it needs to be repeated. Generally advised for deliveries at 24–34 weeks.

Surfactant therapy

Surfactant therapy is given directly down a tracheal tube.

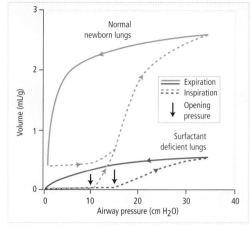

Fig. 27.5 Difference in lung volume for a given airway pressure between normal and surfactant-deficient lungs. If surfactant is present (a) there is a large change in volume for small changes in pressure once the opening pressure is exceeded, and (b) the lungs do not collapse on expiration.

There are two types of surfactant:

• natural surfactants – made from animal lung extracts (bovine or porcine)

• artificial surfactants – manufactured synthetically.

Preterm babies are given surfactant to either prevent or treat RDS (Table 27.1). The two strategies used are:

• prophylactic surfactant for babies at risk of developing RDS

• rescue surfactant therapy once the baby has established RDS.

Systematic reviews and meta-analyses of trials have shown that prophylactic therapy is more effective than rescue treatment.

Table 27.1 Some surfactant preparations.

Name	Source	Dose (mg/kg)	Volume	No. of doses
Survanta (Beractant)	Natural (calf)	100	4 ml	1–4
Curosurf (Poractant)	Natural (porcine)	100–200	1–2 ml	2–3
Infasurf	Natural (calf)	67.5	5 ml	2–3

Prophylaxis – if <30 weeks, surfactant is given in delivery room or on admission to neonatal intensive care unit. Second dose given after 12 hours if required. Sometimes extra doses may be necessary.

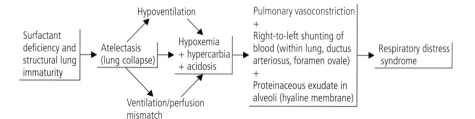

Fig. 27.6 Effect of surfactant deficiency and lung immaturity in preterm infants.

Key points

• Surfactant therapy is a major advance in neonatal care.

• It is most effective when combined with antenatal steroids.

Respiratory distress syndrome (RDS) is:
- also called hyaline membrane disease (HMD) or surfactant deficient lung disease (SDLD)
- the commonest respiratory disorder affecting preterm infants
- a major cause of morbidity and mortality in preterm infants, although this has decreased markedly in recent years.

Risk factors

The predominant risk factor is:
- prematurity (Fig. 28.1), as surfactant is only produced towards the end of the second trimester and early third trimester.
  Other risk factors are:
- maternal diabetes mellitus
- sepsis
- hypoxemia and acidemia
- hypothermia.

Pathology

Characteristic histopathologic features include:
- collapsed terminal air saccules
- overdistended terminal airways
- influx of inflammatory cells into the airway lumen
- interstitial edema and protein leak onto the surface of the airways and air saccules
- hyaline membrane formation in distal and terminal airways (Fig. 28.2)
- necrotic damage to airway epithelial cells.

Pathogenesis

Caused by a deficiency in surfactant production or function. This results in poor lung compliance (i.e. stiff lungs), which in turn leads to alveolar collapse and impaired gas exchange. Lung immaturity may also contribute (see Chapter 27).

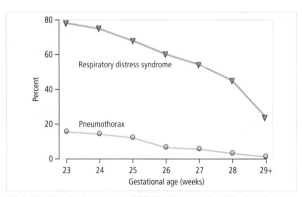

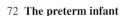

Fig 28.1 Decline in incidence of RDS with gestation. The incidence of pneumothorax is also shown. (NICHD Neonatal Research Network 1997–2000.)

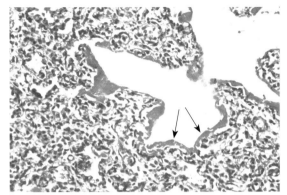

Fig. 28.2 Histology showing characteristic features. The hyaline membrane is shown (arrows).

Key point

Antenatal corticosteroids reduce:
- incidence of respiratory distress syndrome by 60%
- mortality by 40%.

Clinical features

Onset within 4 hours of birth of respiratory distress:
- tachypnea (>60 breaths/minute)
- chest retractions (sternal and intercostal retractions) (Fig. 28.3)
- nasal flaring
- expiratory grunting
- cyanosis (if severe).

Diagnosis is based on history, physical signs, characteristic chest X-ray (Fig. 28.4) and clinical course.

Other causes of respiratory distress in preterm infants are listed in Table 28.1

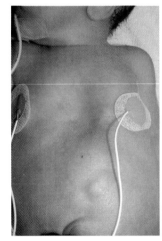

Fig. 28.3 Chest retraction in a preterm infant with respiratory distress.

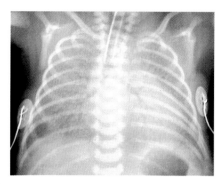

Fig. 28.4 Chest X-ray (after 4 hours of age) in RDS showing:
• diffuse, uniform granular (ground glass) appearance of the lungs from atelectasis
• air bronchogram – outline of air-filled large airways against opaque lungs
• reduced lung volume
• indistinct heart border as the lung fields are opaque ('white-out').
A tracheal tube is in place.

Table 28.1 Causes of respiratory distress in preterm infants.

Common
Respiratory distress syndrome (surfactant deficiency)
Pneumonia/sepsis
Transient tachypnea of the newborn
Uncommon
Pulmonary hypoplasia
Pneumothorax
Congenital heart disease
Rare
Diaphragmatic hernia
Non-respiratory – anemia, hypothermia, metabolic acidosis
Other causes
These are listed in Chapter 38

Natural course

The natural course is for the illness to become worse over the first 24–72 hours and then improve over the next few days. There is initially tissue edema from transudation of fluid into alveoli and subcutaneous tissues, which resolves with improvement of lung disease. These clinical features are markedly ameliorated by antenatal corticosteroids and postnatal surfactant therapy.

Management

This includes:
• antenatal corticosteroids
• surfactant therapy – prophylaxis/rescue via tracheal tube
• oxygen therapy

• prevention of lung collapse – by applying CPAP (continuous positive airway pressure) or PEEP (positive end expiratory pressure) on a mechanical ventilator
• lung expansion – by applying a peak inspiratory pressure with a mechanical ventilator, if necessary
• provision of intensive care (see Chapter 24).

Complications

The main complications are:
• air leaks
• pulmonary hemorrhage
• patent ductus arteriosus
• infection/lung collapse
• intraventricular hemorrhage
• bronchopulmonary dysplasia (chronic lung disease).

Air leaks

Pulmonary interstitial emphysema (PIE)
There is tracking of air from the overdistended terminal airways into the interstitium. Increases risk of pneumothorax and bronchopulmonary dysplasia (chronic lung disease).

Pneumothorax
Occurs in about 10% of infants ventilated for RDS. Presents with:
• increased oxygen requirement
• reduced breath sounds and chest movement on the affected side
• hypoxemia, hypercarbia and acidosis on blood gases
• shock.
  Confirmed by transillumination of the chest or chest X-ray (see Chapter 25).
  A tension pneumothorax is treated by urgent aspiration followed by insertion of a chest tube.
  May occur spontaneously, but is less likely if high airway pressure and asynchrony of the infant's breathing and lung expansion by the ventilator are avoided.

Pulmonary hemorrhage

This is hemorrhagic pulmonary edema. In preterm infants it is usually associated with left heart failure from a patent ductus arteriosus (left-to-right shunting).
  Causes blood staining of tracheal aspirate with or without shock.
  Incidence may be increased to about 2% after surfactant therapy. Coagulation may be deranged.
Treatment:
• increase ventilation and sedation
• surfactant (may be causative and therapeutic)
• replace blood/volume and clotting factors, but avoid fluid overload
• close patent ductus arteriosus.

Hypothermia

Temperature regulation is fundamental to neonatal care.

Hypothermia can cause:

- increased oxygen and energy consumption, resulting in hypoxia, metabolic acidosis and hypoglycemia
- apnea
- neonatal cold injury – redness of the skin from dissociation of hemoglobin
- reduced blood coagulability
- failure to gain weight
- increased mortality.

Newborn babies are particularly liable to hypothermia as:

- they have a large surface area relative to their mass, so there is an imbalance between heat generation (related to mass) and heat loss (surface area)
- their skin is thin and permeable to heat
- they have little subcutaneous fat for insulation
- they have a limited capacity to generate heat as they mainly rely on non-shivering thermogenesis using a special form of adipose tissue, brown fat, which is distributed in the neck, between the scapulae and surrounding the kidneys and adrenals
- their ability to produce heat from sympathetic responses is poor – shivering occurs only at an ambient temperature of <16°C in term infants and does not occur in preterm infants until 2 weeks of age
- preterm infants are unable to curl up to reduce skin exposure.

Evaporative heat loss in preterm infants

Transepidermal water loss:

- is markedly increased in very premature infants (Fig. 29.2a)
- is increased by radiant warmers, phototherapy (unless cold light source) and if the skin is denuded
- is reduced by postnatal age, as the skin thickens
- is reduced by humidity (Fig. 29.2b).

Neutral thermal environment

Infants should be nursed in the neutral thermal environment (Fig. 29.3), and have a core body temperature of 37°C.

Keeping neonates warm

If extremely premature or ill and needs to be naked for observation/procedures:

- place in isolette (incubator) or under radiant warmer
- intensive care unit kept at 26–28°C and draft-free
- use warm, humidified ventilator gases
- clothe with boots and hat (important as the surface area of babies' heads are large relative to their bodies).

How newborn infants lose heat

Convection (Fig. 29.1a)

Determined by:

- temperature difference between skin and air
- area of skin exposed to the air
- movement of surrounding air.

Is an important cause of heat loss, minimized by:

- clothing the infant
- raising temperature of ambient air
- avoiding drafts.

Radiation (Fig. 29.1b)

Depends on temperature difference between skin and surrounding surfaces, i.e. walls of isolette (incubator) or, if under radiant warmer, windows and walls of room; is independent of the air temperature.

Reduced in isolettes (incubators) by having a double wall.

Evaporation (Fig. 29.1c)

Important:

- at birth, when skin is wet – the infant must be dried and wrapped in a warm towel
- in preterm infants, as their skin is very thin and water-permeable
- from the respiratory tree with artificial ventilation/nasal CPAP unless air/oxygen is warm and humidified.

Conduction (Fig. 29.1d)

Loss is small as babies are on mattresses.

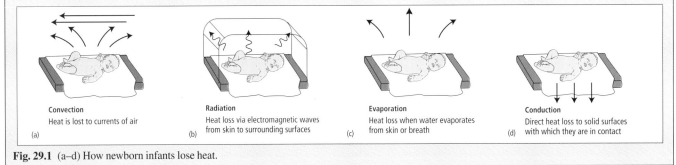

Convection
Heat is lost to currents of air
(a)

Radiation
Heat loss via electromagnetic waves from skin to surrounding surfaces
(b)

Evaporation
Heat loss when water evaporates from skin or breath
(c)

Conduction
Direct heat loss to solid surfaces with which they are in contact
(d)

Fig. 29.1 (a–d) How newborn infants lose heat.

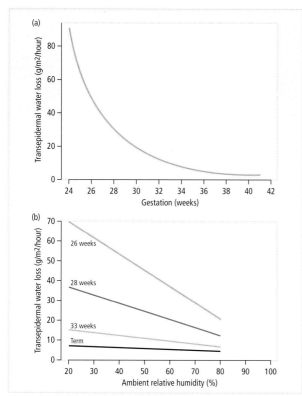

Fig. 29.2 (a) Transepidermal water loss increases with decreasing gestation. (b) Transepidermal water loss is reduced by humidity. (From Hammerlund *et al*. Transepidermal water loss in newborn infants. *Acta Paediatr Scand* 1983; **72**: 721–8.)

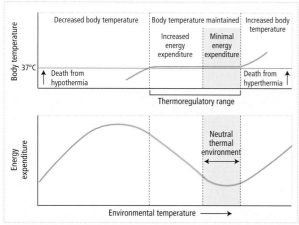

Fig. 29.3 The neutral thermal environment is the temperature range where the heat production is at the minimum needed to maintain normal body temperature. It depends on birthweight and postnatal age and whether the infant is clothed or naked.

If premature but stable:
- clothe
- place in isolette (incubator) or heated mattress in crib/cot
- wrap, keep in a warm, draft-free room.

Isolettes (incubators)

Advantages
- Provide constant, warm environment, even when doors are open.
- Can minimize transepidermal water loss – with high relative humidity.
- Can reduce radiant heat loss if cover the baby and the isolette has double walls.

Disadvantages
- Reduced access for procedures.
- May inhibit parental interaction.
- Noise from isolette's motor and doors.

Radiant warmers

Advantages
- Ease of access for observation and procedures.
- Rapid increase in temperature.

Disadvantages
- High transepidermal water loss makes fluid balance problematical.
- Difficult to provide extra humidity – partially achieved by covering the infant with cling film, insulating material, etc., and giving extra humidity.
- High convective heat losses.

Combined isolettes (incubators) with inbuilt radiant warmers

Radiant heat is used only when access is required, e.g. for procedures.

Key point

A normal core temperature does not mean a neutral thermal environment – it may be achieved by thermal stress.

Question

When are heated mattresses useful?

They allow some stable preterm infants to be nursed in a crib (cot) instead of an isolette (incubator). Also to warm infants who have become cold, or in the operating room, during imaging studies or transport.

30 Growth and nutrition

Growth

Between 24 and 36 weeks' gestation, a fetus growing along the 50th centile gains 15 g/kg/day. Infants who are fed enterally require 120–140 kcal/kg/day to maintain this rate of growth. As these high energy requirements often cannot be met, the weight of extremely preterm infants is often initially static or may decline, and the infant may take up to 21 days to regain birth weight. Thereafter, their growth improves but is often suboptimal (Fig. 30.1). The reason for this growth failure includes:

- the infant is unable to tolerate high volumes of nutrients
- fluids may be restricted, e.g. patent ductus arteriosus
- intercurrent illness, e.g. infection.

Nutrition

Which milk?

Breast milk

Is the milk of choice. Advantages over formula feeds (also see Chapter 19) are:

- better tolerated
- associated with a lower incidence of necrotizing enterocolitis and provides some protection against infection
- contains hormones and growth factors
- has better absorption of fats and improved bioavailability of trace minerals
- promotes mother–infant bonding
- it is associated with improved cognitive development later in childhood.

Disadvantages are:

- depends on the mother being able to express sufficient milk over a prolonged period.
- growth of the preterm infant may be suboptimal. Breast milk may need to be enhanced with a human milk fortifier to increase its energy, protein and mineral content. Human milk fortifiers contain cow's milk protein. Fortification is usually stopped once the infant is entirely breast-fed or weighs more than 2 kg.

Low birthweight infant formulas

These have been developed to supply the increased energy (24 kcal/

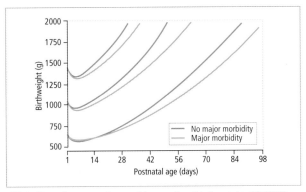

Fig. 30.1 Growth curves observed in very low birthweight (VLBW) infants according to birthweight, with and without major morbidities. (From Ehrenkranz *et al. Pediatrics* 1999; **104**: 280.)

oz, 80 kcal/100 ml), protein, sodium, calcium and phosphate required by low birthweight infants (Table 30.1).

Supplements

- **Iron** is given to all preterm infants once they are on full enteral feeds and are not receiving blood transfusions. Supplementation is usually continued for six months to one year.
- **Multivitamins** (A, B_{12}, C, D and E) are given routinely. Folic acid is given in some centers.
- **Vitamin K** is given to all infants, including the preterm, as prophylaxis against hemorrhagic disease of the newborn.

Feeding

Whereas the healthy newborn term infant can be put to the breast shortly after birth, extremely preterm infants cannot feed for themselves as they:

- are unable to suck and swallow until about 34–35 weeks of gestation (Figs 30.2–4)
- are initially unable to tolerate milk in sufficient quantity to meet their nutritional requirements.

A number of strategies are adopted to overcome these problems.

Table 30.1 Composition of various milks.

	Cow's milk	Mature term breast milk	Preterm breast milk	Fortified preterm breast	Low birth-weight formula	Term formula
Energy (kcal/100 ml)	67	70	67	74	80	66
Carbohydrate (g/100 ml)	4.6	7	6	–	8.5	6.9
Fat (g/100 ml)	3.9	4.2	4	4	4.4	3.6
Protein (g/100 ml)	3.4	1.3	1.8–2.4	3.7	2.2	1.5
Na (mmol/L)	22	7	22	31	13–20	8
K (mmol/L)	39	15	18	–	18	17
Ca (mmol/L)	30	9	6	27	18–27	12–20
Phosphate (mmol/L)	30	5	5	38	11–17	12–18

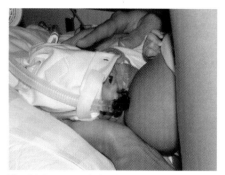

Fig. 30.2 Preterm infant learning to suck at the breast whilst still on continuous positive airway pressure (CPAP).

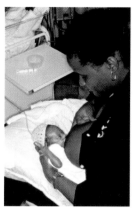

Fig. 30.3 Preterm infant learning to breast feed whilst still receiving nasogastric gavage (tube) feeds

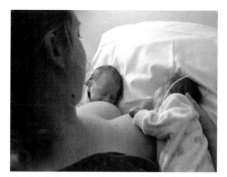

Fig. 30.4 Preterm twins successfully learning to feed at the breast.

Minimal enteral (non-nutritive) feeding

A small volume (e.g. 10–20 ml/kg/day), preferably with expressed breast milk, is given initially to stimulate gut hormone production. This helps intestinal maturation, motility and gall bladder function, decreasing the time taken to establish full enteral feeding; and lowers serum bilirubin concentrations. Feeding is introduced particularly slowly in infants who are growth-restricted and have reversed end-diastolic blood flow velocity on antenatal Doppler ultrasound because of the increased risk of necrotizing enterocolitis.

Gavage (tube) feeding

Used when infants are too immature (<34 weeks' gestational age) or ill to feed for themselves but are able to tolerate enteral feeds. The volume of milk is gradually increased. Feeds are withheld if aspirates are more than half the volume given or if bilious with abdominal distension, blood in the stool or other features suggesting necrotizing enterocolitis. Reduced gut motility in very low birthweight infants may necessitate suppositories for constipation.

The tube may be orogastric or nasogastric. As nasogastric tubes lie in the narrowest part of the upper airway, just behind the nose, a size 5 French gauge tube increases airway resistance by 30–50% in preterm infants. This increases the work of breathing and may increase the frequency of apnea. Some units avoid nasogastric tubes if less than 35 weeks' gestation, but orogastric tubes are more difficult to fix securely.

There is conflicting evidence regarding continuous versus bolus feeding in relation to weight gain and the incidence of apnea and bradycardia. The infant's oxygen tension falls with feeds in both preterm and term infants. It has been argued that continuous feeding is more physiologic for preterm infants because it is a closer approximation to the way a fetus is fed *in utero*. However, bolus feeds are preferred as the response of gut hormones is more physiologic.

Total parenteral nutrition (TPN)

A mixture of carbohydrate, protein, fat, vitamins and trace elements allows nutrition to be provided whilst oral feeding is established. It is usually given via a central venous line but may be given peripherally. It is associated with a number of complications:

- line-related infection
- conjugated hyperbilirubinemia
- electrolyte disorders
- hyperglycemia
- chemical burns from extravasation
- pleural or pericardial effusion – if central line lies in the heart.

Volume of fluids

A guide to average total fluid intake is shown in Table 30.2. It is adjusted according to plasma electrolytes, creatinine, acid–base status and the infant's weight, all of which are measured regularly over the first few days. It is markedly affected by:

- gestational age
- thermal environment (radiant warmer or isolette)
- evaporative water loss (reduced by humidity, etc.).

Once the preterm infant is stable and on full enteral feeds, electrolytes, creatinine and phosphate, calcium and alkaline phosphatase can be checked weekly.

Table 30.2 Typical fluid intake according to postnatal age.

Postnatal age	Fluid intake (ml/kg/24 h)	
	<2.5 kg	>2.5 kg
Day 1	60–100	40–80
Day 2	90–120	60–100
Day 3	120–150	90–120
Day 4	150	120–150
Days 5 and over	150–180	150

These are the most common causes of acquired brain injury in premature infants. Their incidence is inversely related to gestational age.

- **Hemorrhage** – occurs in 25–30% of VLBW (very low birthweight) infants. Involves the germinal matrix, an immature capillary network, which overlies the head of the caudate nucleus. The hemorrhage may be confined to the germinal matrix, may extend into the ventricle or involve the parenchyma. Hemorrhagic parenchymal lesions are thought to be mainly venous infarcts from impaired venous drainage. Hemorrhage usually occurs within 72 hours of birth. The germinal matrix disappears at about 32 weeks gestation, so hemorrhage is uncommon beyond this gestation.
- **Periventricular leukomalacia (PVL)** – loss of periventricular white matter in watershed areas around the lateral ventricles from hypoxia–ischemia. Probably most occur before birth, but some occur postnatally. Only becomes evident as cystic lesions on ultrasound 3 or more weeks after the insult. Cystic PVL is detectable on ultrasound in 3% of VLBW infants; less severe damage is represented by a persistent flare (echodensity) in the periventricular white matter.

The appearance of these lesions on cranial ultrasound is shown in Chapter 75.

Diagnosis

This is by cranial ultrasound at the bedside (Table 31.2). In very low birthweight (VLBW) infants, it is performed shortly after birth to identify antenatal lesions, during the first week of life to identify hemorrhages and repeated periodically to identify and monitor hydrocephalus and appearance of periventricular leukomalacia (PVL).

Ultrasound is excellent for detecting hemorrhage and ventricular dilatation, but is relatively insensitive in detecting white matter damage. MRI when older is more sensitive than ultrasound for white matter injury.

Pathogenesis (Figs 31.1 and 31.2) and incidence (Table 31.1)

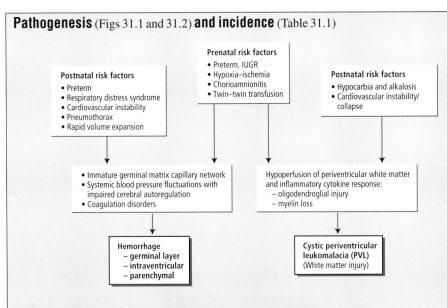

Fig. 31.1 Pathogenesis of cerebral hemorrhage and cystic periventricular leukomalacia (PVL).

Question

What is meant by cerebral autoregulation?

It is the maintenance of cerebral blood flow over a wide range in blood pressure.

This blood pressure range is narrow in preterm infants; there is cerebral hypoperfusion accompanying falls in blood pressure, leading to hemorrhage or ischemic damage.

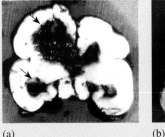
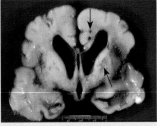

(a)   (b)

Fig. 31.2 Autopsy specimen showing (a) large parenchymal and intraventricular hemorrhage and (b) ventricular dilatation and cystic periventricular leukomalacia (PVL).

Key point

There has been a marked reduction in the incidence of post-hemorrhagic hydrocephalus requiring shunts.

Table 31.1 Incidence of hemorrhage or periventricular leukomalacia (PVL) by birthweight.

Birthweight (grams)	Hemorrhage (all grades)	PVL
501–750	46%	5%
751–1000	32%	4%
1001–1250	21%	3%
1251–1500	16%	2%
	Severe (Grade III/IV)	
<1500	10%	3%

Vermont–Oxford Network, 2004.

Table 31.2 A classification of lesions identified on intracranial ultrasound.

Hemorrhage
  Grade I – Isolated germinal matrix hemorrhage
  Grade II – Intraventricular hemorrhage without ventricular dilatation
  Grade III – Intraventricular hemorrhage with acute ventricular dilatation
  Grade IV – Parenchymal hemorrhagic venous infarct
Periventricular leukomalacia (PVL)
  Cysts – localized and small or widespread
  Porencephalic cyst – single, large cyst
Ventricular dilatation

Clinical features

Most infants are asymptomatic. Clinical features include:
- increased ventilatory support
- abnormal neurologic signs including seizures
- apnea and bradycardia
- shock.

Laboratory findings

Mostly not specifically attributable to cerebral hemorrhage. May include:
- acute anemia
- hyperglycemia
- unexplained, severe metabolic acidosis
- hyperkalemia
- electrolyte imbalance
- coagulation abnormalities.

Key point

Don't overestimate the long-term significance of minor abnormalities on cranial ultrasound.

Management

- Optimize:
  – airway and breathing – provide oxygenation/ventilation as needed; avoid hypo- or hypercarbia
  – circulation – maintain adequate intravascular volume and blood pressure
  – sedation/analgesia – avoid unnecessary manipulation of infant.
- Treat seizures.
- Correct significant coagulation abnormalities.
- Monitor complications – hydrocephalus.

Prognosis

- Small germinal matrix or intraventricular hemorrhage – similar to normal ultrasound.
- Large parenchymal hemorrhage/large porencephalic cyst/hydrocephalus needing shunt – appreciable mortality, high risk of cerebral palsy and learning difficulties.
- Localized cysts/persistent flares – normal or mild spastic diplegia.
- Widespread cysts – all have cerebral palsy, usually spastic diplegia or quadriplegia with or without learning difficulties.

Prevention

- Avoid delivery before 30 weeks of gestation unless essential, and give antenatal corticosteroids.
- Avoid perinatal hypoxia–ischemia.
- Efficient resuscitation.
- Optimize intensive care – especially ventilation and circulation.
  Giving the infant indomethacin prophylactically reduces the incidence of severe hemorrhage but does not improve neurodevelopmental outcome.

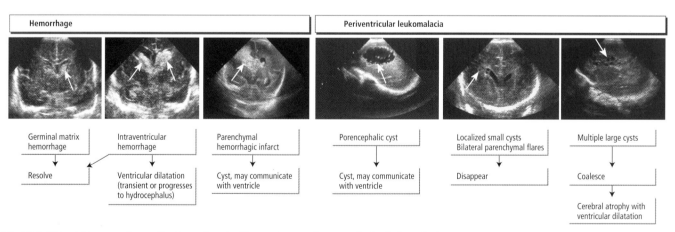

Fig. 31.3 Natural history and complications of cerebral hemorrhage and periventricular leukomalacia.

32 Patent ductus arteriosus (PDA)

Normal infants

Ductus arteriosus – connects the pulmonary artery with the descending aorta (Fig. 32.1).

In utero – ductal patency

This is dependent on low PaO_2 and high concentrations of vasodilating prostaglandins (PGE_2 and PGI_2).

Postnatal – ductal constriction

This is promoted by:
- the rise in oxygen tension with the first breaths
- the increase in pulmonary blood flow, which enhances clearance of the local vasodilating prostaglandins.

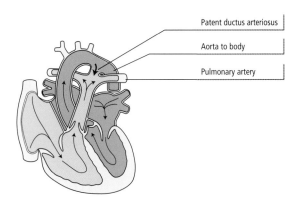

Fig. 32.1 Anatomy of the ductus arteriosus, with left to right flow across it.

Clinical features

- Tachypnea.
- Increase in oxygen requirement.
- Carbon dioxide retention, difficulty weaning from mechanical ventilation.
- Apnea and bradycardia.
- Tachycardia.
- Widened pulse pressure, causing bounding pulses.
- Active precordium.
- Heart murmur (see below).
- Hepatomegaly (from right-sided heart failure).

Heart murmur
Characteristic cardiac murmur (Fig. 32.2):
- systolic
- best heard at left sternal border.

If heart failure is present:
- gallop rhythm (extra third heart sound)
- may be loud pulmonic component (P_2) of second heart sound
  Silent PDA, i.e. no murmur but PDA present – common, usually large shunt.

  The classic continuous murmur – in systole and extending into diastole – that is heard in older infants is rarely present in preterm infants.

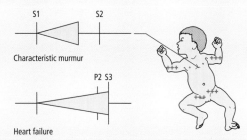

Fig. 32.2 Cardiac murmur and bounding pulses from shunting across a patent ductus arteriosus.

Investigations
CHEST X-RAY (Fig. 32.3)

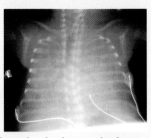

Fig. 32.3 Chest X-ray showing increased pulmonary vasculature markings and cardiomegaly. But often unhelpful diagnostically.

ECHOCARDIOGRAPHY WITH PULSED COLOR DOPPLER
- Confirms the diagnosis.
- Provides details of size and direction of the shunt and its hemodynamic consequences.

Echocardiographic diagnosis:
- Direct visualization – diameter (>1.5 mm), direction of shunt.
- Left atrial enlargement (left atrial:aortic root ratio >1.5:1).
- Absent or retrograde diastolic flow in postductal aorta.

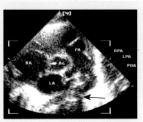

Fig. 32.4 Visualization of a patent ductus arteriosus (arrow).

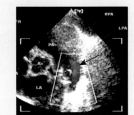

Fig. 32.5 Pulsed color Doppler showing shunting across the ductus arteriosus (arrow).

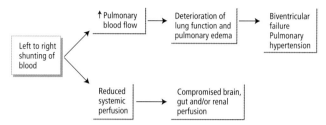

Fig. 32.6 Physiologic consequences of a patent ductus arteriosus

Ductal closure takes place in two steps:
- functional closure – 24–48 hours after birth
- anatomic closure – may take 2–3 weeks.

Ductal closure

In preterm infants, there may be delay in anatomic closure. Blood flows left to right across the patent ductus, from the higher systemic blood pressure to the low pulmonary artery pressure (Fig. 32.6). However, in respiratory distress syndrome, pulmonary artery pressure is increased and the shunt may be bidirectional or right to left.

In term infants, a patent ductus arteriosus is a permanent defect in the muscle wall of the duct and is unlikely to close spontaneously.

Risk factors

- Prematurity – incidence increases with decreasing gestational age; most are less than 32 weeks' gestational age.
- Respiratory distress syndrome.
- Fluid overload.
- Sepsis.

Management
Medical management

Aim is to control heart failure and close the duct pharmacologically.

It consists of:
- fluid restriction (usually 100 ml/kg/day)
- diuretics may be given for heart failure
- prostaglandin synthase inhibitors, also called cyclooxygenase inhibitors (COXi):
  – indomethacin
  – ibuprofen.

Indomethacin has been widely used for many years. More recently ibuprofen has been introduced. It has similar efficacy but, in contrast to indomethacin, there is less reduction in cerebral, renal and mesenteric blood flow. Other side effects and contraindications are shown in Table 32.1. Indomethacin may be given as a short course in high dosage or a longer course in lower dosage. The duct closes in >60% after a single course, but often remains patent and further courses are required.

Surgical closure

Performed if medical treatment fails.

Video-assisted thoracoscopic surgery (VATS) is now available in some centers, avoiding the need for a thoracotomy.

Complications of surgery are:
- recurrent laryngeal nerve damage
- chylothorax from damage to thoracic duct
- pneumothorax
- ligation of pulmonary artery by mistake
- mortality (<1%).

Complications

These include:
- pulmonary hemorrhage
- cranial hemorrhage
- necrotizing enterocolitis
- bronchopulmonary dysplasia (chronic lung disease).

Table 32.1 Indomethacin and ibuprofen.

Side effects	Contraindications
Decrease platelet aggregation, may worsen bleeding	Abnormal renal function with oliguria
Gastrointestinal bleeding	Thrombocytopenia (platelet count <75 000/mm^3 (<75 × 10^9/L)
	Gastrointestinal bleeding

Infection

In preterm infants, infection is a major cause of morbidity and mortality.

Preterm infants are especially vulnerable because:
• they have reduced cellular and humoral immunity – this is because IgG antibodies are transferred from mother to fetus mainly during the third trimester
• their skin is thin and readily denuded by skin electrodes, catheters and tape, providing a portal of entry and a site of colonization for organisms
• central venous catheters and tracheal tubes are left in place for prolonged periods and are a potential focus for infection
• cross-infection is readily spread from infant to infant in neonatal nurseries on the hands of staff and from contaminated equipment.

Early-onset infection (<72 hours)

Acquired before birth from chorioamnionitis or maternal bacteremia or from the birth canal.

The most common organisms are Group B streptococci and coliforms.

Late-onset sepsis (>72 hours)

Mainly due to nosocomial (hospital-acquired) infection. The most common cause is coagulase-negative staphylococcus (CONS). Other organisms are shown in Fig. 33.1.

There is marked variation in nosocomial infection rates among units. This results in wide variation in infection-related morbidity, duration of hospitalization, cost and mortality.

Fungal infections

In very low birthweight infants:
• incidence 1–10%
• mortality (up to 35%).

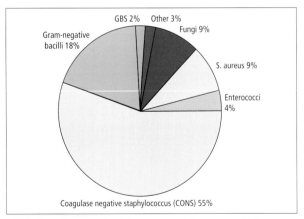

Fig. 33.1 Organisms causing late-onset sepsis in very low birthweight infants. (NICHD Neonatal Network. *J Pediatr* 1996; 129:63.)

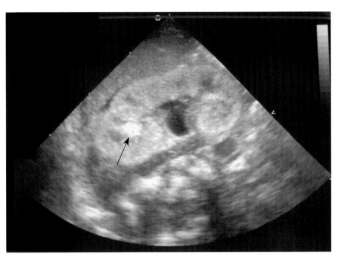

Fig. 33.2 Fungal ball in the kidney from *Candida* sepsis on renal ultrasound.

Candida albicans is the most common organism (Fig. 33.2). The source of infection is colonization of the gastrointestinal tract. Oral and topical antifungal agents are often given as prophylaxis to infants receiving prolonged antibiotic therapy, although this practice is not uniformly accepted.

Treatment is with amphotericin B or flucytosine.

Presentation and management

These are described in Chapter 40.

Jaundice

Most preterm infants develop jaundice from unconjugated hyperbilirubinemia in the first week of life. The level of bilirubin that is potentially damaging is lower than in more mature infants. The bilirubin peaks at around day 5 of life and should be closely monitored.

Conjugated hyperbilirubinemia is mainly associated with total parenteral nutrition (TPN), necrotizing enterocolitis and congenital infection. Management is described in Chapter 39.

Anemia

Common in VLBW (very low birthweight) infants, mainly because of:
• blood loss from repeated blood sampling and the preterm infant's small blood volume of only 80 ml/kg
• physiologic anemia of prematurity. This occurs at 2–4 months of age due to:
  – low red cell mass
  – shortened red cell survival
  – markedly increased requirements from growth.

Treatment

Blood transfusions

Aim is to restore or maintain adequate tissue oxygen delivery, but as there are no reliable symptoms or signs to determine this, the indications in neonates are controversial (Table 33.1). Kept to a minimum because of potential hazards. Splitting adult donor bags to allow several transfusions from the same donor reduces potential risks by reducing number of donors.

Oral iron therapy

Given to prevent anemia of prematurity, unless the infant has received a recent blood transfusion.

Oral folic acid

Given in some centers.

Osteopenia of prematurity

Metabolic bone disease may occur at several weeks of age, causing:
- reduced bone mineralization with widening and cupping of the wrists, knees and ribs on X-ray, as with rickets (Fig. 33.3)
- failure in linear growth
- pathologic fractures, particularly of ribs and long bones (Fig. 33.4).

Investigations show:
- calcium – normal or raised
- phosphate – low
- alkaline phosphatase (a marker of bone turnover) – markedly raised.

Osteopenia of prematurity is due to phosphorus deficiency from urinary loss and increased requirements.

It can be prevented by providing additional phosphate in total parenteral nutrition, by fortifying expressed breast milk or by giving oral phosphate to maintain age-appropriate plasma phosphate levels. It can be problematic to provide sufficient phosphate for infants requiring total parenteral nutrition for a prolonged period.

Treatment is with sodium or potassium acid phosphate and vitamin D supplements.

Table 33.1 Indications for blood transfusions in preterm infants (College of American Pathologists, 1998).

Acute blood loss with shock
Hb <12 g/dl – if in oxygen with mechanical ventilation, congenital heart disease with cyanosis or heart failure
Hb <10 g/dl – if moderate oxygen requirement via nasal cannula
Hb <8 g/dl – if apnea and bradycardia, sustained tachycardia, failure to gain weight, mild oxygen requirement
Hb <7 g/dl and reticulocyte count <100 000/ml – even if asymptomatic

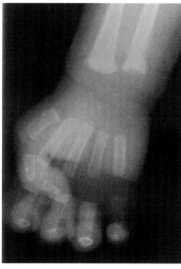

Fig. 33.3 Reduced bone mineralization with widening and cupping of the wrist bones from osteopenia of prematurity.

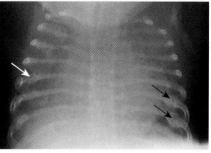

Fig. 33.4 Rib fractures (arrows) and reduced bone mineralization from osteopenia of prematurity. (Courtesy of Dr Richard Nicholl.)

Apnea, bradycardia and desaturations

Common in VLBW (very low birthweight) infants.

Definition (Fig. 34.1)
Inter-relationship between apnea, bradycardia and desaturation is complex, so monitor not only respiration but also heart rate and saturation.

Hypoxemia with bradycardia is harmful if prolonged.

Classification
- **Central** – cessation of chest wall motion due to loss of respiratory neural output.
- **Obstructive** – persistence of obstructed inspiratory efforts throughout the apnea with no airflow. Rare, unless associated with neck flexion. Presents with bradycardia with or without desaturation. May not be detected on standard clinical impedance respiratory monitor as they detect chest wall movement as a breath, although there is no airflow.
- **Mixed** – most common; a combination of both of above, with obstructed inspiratory efforts intermittently throughout the apnea.

Episodes of desaturation
- May accompany short (5–10 seconds) respiratory pauses, especially if baseline SaO_2 is low.
- During assisted ventilation they are secondary to hypoventilation.
- Variable relationship with bradycardia.

Causes
Usually due to prematurity – must consider or exclude:
- infection (most common)
- necrotizing enterocolitis
- heart failure – patent ductus arteriosus, etc.
- hypoglycemia, electrolyte abnormality
- inborn error of metabolism
- anemia
- seizures.

Treatment
Most apneic spells are brief and self-limiting.

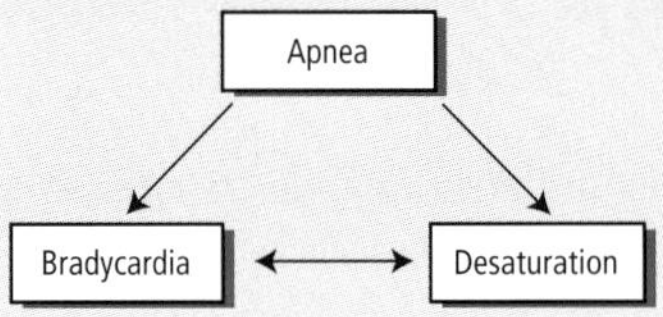

Fig. 34.1 Apnea is absence of breathing for more than 10–15 seconds and may result in bradycardia and/or desaturation.

If not:
- Check airway.
- Gentle tactile stimulation.
- Nasal CPAP (continuous positive airway pressure) – very effective, eliminates obstructive apnea.
- Methylxanthines – caffeine or theophylline. Caffeine more widely used as fewer side-effects and drug level monitoring not needed.
- Mechanical ventilation.

Prognosis
Apnea and bradycardia continue in some preterm infants beyond 36 weeks of gestational age, particularly in association with bronchopulmonary dysplasia (chronic lung disease), but rarely beyond 43–44 weeks. Continue to hospitalize if symptomatic apnea and bradycardia until absent for several days. Not a risk factor for SIDS (sudden infant death syndrome).

Question
What is the relationship of apnea to feeding?
Hypoventilation, apnea and even cyanosis commonly accompany onset of oral (especially bottle) feeds.

These episodes of hypoventilation typically resolve rapidly without the need for further intervention.

Gastroesophageal reflux and apnea are both common in preterm infants, but rarely temporally related.

Pharmacologic treatment of reflux often fails to abolish apnea.

Retinopathy of prematurity (ROP)

Eye disease of prematurity. Highest incidence in extremely low birthweight infants.

Hyperoxia causes retinal vasoconstriction which acts as a stimulus for inappropriate and excessive growth of retinal vessels. This is mediated by vascular endothelial growth factor (VEGF).

Keeping preterm infants in inappropriately high oxygen concentrations results in a high incidence of ROP, causing blindness (see Chapter 64). However, in VLBW (very low birthweight) infants, even with oxygenation closely monitored (attempting to keep PaO_2

at 50–80 mmHg, i.e. 6.5–10.5 kPa, oxygen saturation 88–95%), about 40% develop ROP, with 5% needing treatment and 1% have severe visual impairment.

Visual outcome also depends on associated neurologic injury, myopia and squint.

ROP causes 3–10% of childhood visual impairment in developed countries.

Screening

Preterm infants are screened selectively (Table 34.1). Findings are

Table 34.1 Screening for retinopathy of prematurity.

	US	UK
Who?	Birth: <1500 g or <29 weeks	Birth: <1501 g and <32 weeks
When?	4–6 weeks' chronological age or 31–33 weeks' postmenstrual age, whichever is later	6–7 weeks' chronological age
Follow up?	Until retinopathy shows signs of regression or until 36 weeks' postmenstrual age if no disease	

classified according to the stage of advancement and the zone affected (Table 34.2 and Fig. 34.2).

Treatment

Stage 1 or 2 disease resolves spontaneously. Plus disease requires laser therapy (Fig. 34.6).

Table 34.2 International classification of retinopathy of prematurity (revised 2005).

Stage 1 – Flat demarcation line between normally vascularized and non-vascularized retina (Fig. 34.3)
Stage 2 – Demarcation line extends off the retina as a ridge
Stage 3 – New vessels behind the ridge with or without vitreous hemorrhage (extraretinal fibrovascular proliferation) (Fig. 34.4)
Stage 4 – Partial retinal detachment
Stage 5 – Total retinal detachment (Fig. 34.5)
Plus disease – active progressive disease
Pre-plus disease – abnormal dilatation and tortuosity of posterior pole vessels
Aggressive posterior ROP – rapidly progressing, severe form

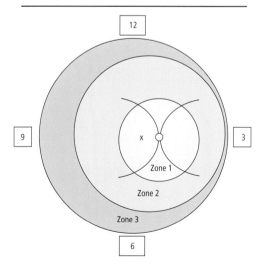

Fig. 34.2 Zones of retina. Numbers at the periphery indicate clock hour.

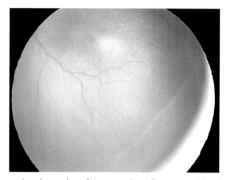

Fig. 34.3 Stage 1 retinopathy of prematurity. (Courtesy of Prof. Alistair Fielder.)

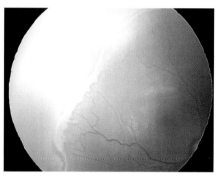

Fig. 34.4 Stage 3 retinopathy of prematurity in a Black-African infant. (Courtesy of Prof. Alistair Fielder.)

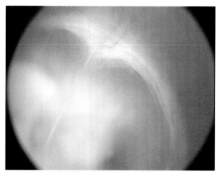

Fig. 34.5 Stage 5 retinopathy of prematurity showing retinal detachment.

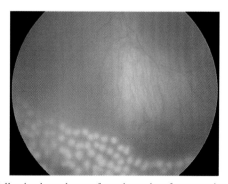

Fig. 34.6 Following laser therapy for retinopathy of prematurity.

Apnea, bradycardia and desaturations, retinopathy of prematurity 85

Necrotizing enterocolitis (NEC) is the most serious abdominal disorder of preterm infants. It occurs in 2–10% of VLBW (very low birthweight) infants and has a mortality of 25–30%.

The incidence increases with decreasing gestational age; it is rare in term infants. It is a syndrome characterized by abdominal distension, bilious aspirates, bloody stools and intramural air (*pneumatosis intestinalis*) on abdominal X-ray.

There is inflammation of the bowel wall, which may progress to necrosis and perforation. It may involve a localized section of bowel (most often the terminal ileum) or be generalized.

Cases may be sporadic or sometimes occur in epidemics.

Risk factors

Pathogenesis is unknown, but several risk factors have been identified (Fig. 35.1).

Laboratory findings

These include:
- raised acute-phase reactant (C-reactive protein, CRP)
- thrombocytopenia
- neutropenia, neutrophilia
- anemia
- blood culture positive
- coagulation abnormalities
- metabolic acidosis
- hypoxia, hypercapnia
- hyponatremia, hyperkalemia
- increased BUN (blood urea)
- hyperbilirubinemia.

Radiologic abnormalities

- Dilated loops of bowel.
- Thickened intestinal wall.
- Inspissated stool (mottled appearance).
- Intramural air (*pneumatosis intestinalis*) (Fig. 35.3).

Clinical features

Onset is at 1–2 weeks but may be up to several weeks of age, with:
- bilious aspirates/vomiting
- feeding intolerance
- bloody stools
- abdominal distention and tenderness (Fig. 35.2), which may progress to perforation (Table 35.1).
- features of sepsis:
  - temperature instability
  - jaundice
  - apnea and bradycardia
  - lethargy
  - hypoperfusion, shock.

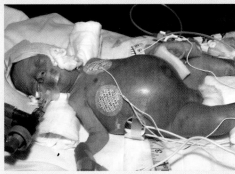

Fig. 35.2 Abdominal distension and shiny abdominal skin in necrotizing enterocolitis.

Table 35.1 Clinical signs of peritonitis/perforation.

Abdominal tenderness
Guarding
Tense, discolored abdominal wall
Abdominal wall edema
Absent bowel sounds
Abdominal mass

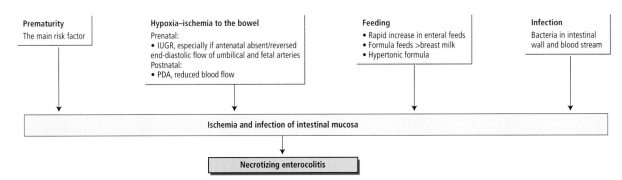

Fig. 35.1 Risk factors in the pathogenesis of necrotizing enterocolitis.

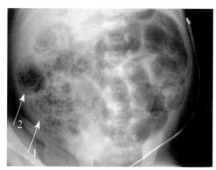

Fig. 35.3 Abdominal X-ray showing dilated loops of bowel, inspissated stool (arrow 1) and intramural air (arrow 2). (Courtesy of Dr Annemarie Jeanes.)

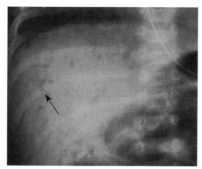

Fig. 35.4 Air in portal venous system (arrow). (Courtesy of Dr Annemarie Jeanes.)

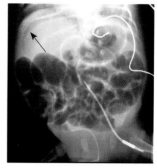

Fig. 35.5 Bowel perforation showing air under the diaphragm (arrow) and outlining the falciform ligament. (Courtesy of Dr Annemarie Jeanes.)

- Air in portal venous system (Fig. 35.4).
- Bowel perforation:
  - gasless abdomen/ascites
  - pneumoperitoneum
  - air below diaphragm/around the falciform ligament (Fig. 35.5).

Management (Table 35.2)

Table 35.2 Management of necrotizing enterocolitis.

Treatment	Rationale/goals
Secure airway and breathing	Maintain adequate oxygenation and ventilation
	Abdominal distension may compromise breathing
Circulation	
• establish vascular access	Infusion of fluids
• give intravascular volume replacement (saline, blood, fresh frozen plasma)	Treat hypoperfusion/hypovolemic shock
• correct metabolic acidosis	Improve organ and tissue perfusion
Place large-bore naso/orogastric tube	Intestinal decompression, bowel rest
NPO (nil by mouth) – start parenteral nutrition	Support nutritional demands for growth
Broad-spectrum antibiotics	Gram-positive, -negative and anaerobic coverage
	Consider antifungal agents
Treat coagulopathy (fresh frozen plasma, platelets, cryoprecipitate)	Avoid bleeding complications
Monitor regularly – clinical, radiographic and laboratory investigations	Necrotizing enterocolitis can worsen very quickly
Surgery	Indications – bowel perforation or failure to resolve on medical treatment
Options are:	
• peritoneal drainage at bedside	
• laparotomy – resection of non-viable bowel and anastomosis or ileostomy or colostomy	

Sequelae

Short term

These are:
- electrolyte depletion.
- complications of prolonged parenteral nutrition – infection, electrolyte derangement, conjugated hyperbilirubinemia, etc.

Long term

Short bowel syndrome:
- diarrhea (from loss of bowel mucosa and rapid gastrointestinal transit)
- growth failure
- vitamin B_{12} deficiency if terminal ileum resected
- stricture formation – causes intestinal obstruction and/or intestinal hemorrhage.

Prevention

- Use breast milk if possible.
- Avoid hyperosmolar feeds.
- Avoid rapid increase in feed volume in very immature infants, especially if intrauterine growth restriction with absent/reverse end-diastolic Doppler waveform antenatally.
- Use of prebiotics and probiotics to maintain normal gut flora is being investigated.

Key point

NEC is often suspected, although all the classic clinical features are not present. Treatment may need to be started whilst awaiting investigation results and before the clinical course becomes evident. Surgical consultation should be initiated early.

Bronchopulmonary dysplasia (BPD, chronic lung disease) is a major cause of morbidity and mortality in preterm infants. It develops in about 37% of very low birthweight infants. The incidence is highest in the extremely preterm (Fig. 36.1). It is uncommon in infants born after 32 weeks' gestational age.

Definition

A consensus conference (NICHD/NHLB/ORD, 2004) recommended definitions based on severity of illness:
- oxygen requirement at 28 days of age (this is used in many trials)
- oxygen requirement and characteristic chest X-ray changes at 28 days
- oxygen requirement at 36 weeks' postmenstrual age. This is increasingly used as it identifies infants most likely to have long-term complications.

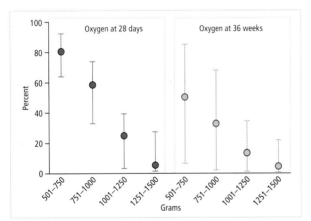

Fig. 36.1 Incidence of bronchopulmonary dysplasia (BPD, chronic lung disease) with confidence intervals by birthweight. (Lemons *et al.* NICHD Neonatal Network.)

It also recommended that the term 'bronchopulmonary dysplasia' be used rather than 'chronic lung disease'.

Predisposing factors

The cause is unknown. It is a multifactorial disorder.

It most often develops in extremely preterm infants with surfactant deficiency or immature lungs who require mechanical ventilation. The higher the pressures and oxygen concentration required and the longer mechanical ventilation is needed, the more likely the infant is to develop BPD. However, some extremely preterm infants with minimal lung disease in the first few days of life develop an increasing and prolonged oxygen requirement. There may be a genetic predisposition – it is more common if there is a family history of reactive airway disease.

Other risk factors are shown in Fig. 36.2.

Clinical features

These are:
- skin pallor
- tachypnea
- hyperexpanded chest
- chest retractions
- auscultation – crackles and wheezes
- fluid retention
- heart failure
- recurrent pneumonia
- growth failure.

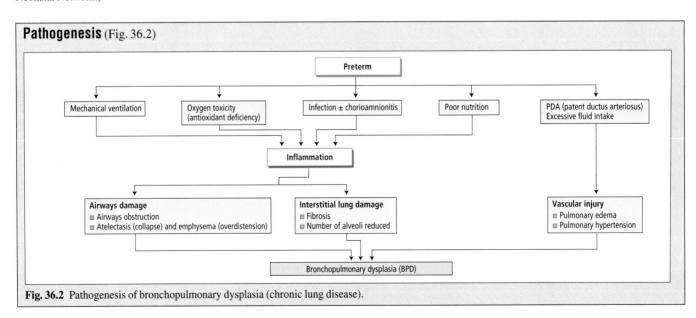

Fig. 36.2 Pathogenesis of bronchopulmonary dysplasia (chronic lung disease).

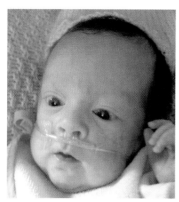

Fig. 36.3 Infant with bronchopulmonary dysplasia receiving low-flow nasal oxygen.

Chest X-ray (Fig. 36.4)

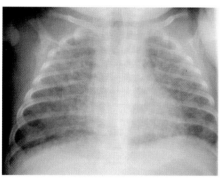

Fig. 36.4 Chest X-ray in bronchopulmonary dysplasia (chronic lung disease) showing lung collapse, fibrosis, cystic changes and overdistention of the lungs.

Management

This is with:
- additional oxygen and respiratory support (mechanical ventilation/nasal CPAP/low flow nasal cannula) to maintain satisfactory oxygenation (SaO$_2$ 88–95%) (Fig. 36.3)
- nutrition:
  - increased caloric requirements (130–150 kcal/kg) because of increased work of breathing
  - delay in establishing feeding
  - gastroesophageal reflux (may result in aspiration)
  - prevention of osteopenia of prematurity with phosphate supplements
- drug therapy:
  - diuretics (transient improvement)
  - inhaled bronchodilators
  - corticosteroid therapy (see below)
  - sedation – may be required for episodes of agitation and desaturation.

Long-term consequences of severe BPD

- Prolonged oxygen therapy over many months. May need to be given at home.
- Feeding problems requiring prolonged nasogastric/gastrostomy feeding.
- Inguinal hernias (from raised intra-abdominal pressure and muscular weakness).
- Risk of RSV (respiratory syncytial virus) infection causing bronchiolitis (may benefit from protection with the monoclonal antibody palivizumab).
- Rehospitalization because of respiratory infection – needing additional oxygen/nasal CPAP (continuous positive airway pressure)/mechanical ventilation.
- Increased risk of neurodevelopmental problems during childhood.
- Rarely, death from acute chest infection or cor pulmonale (pulmonary hypertension).

Strategies for prevention

These include:
- antenatal corticosteroids.
- surfactant therapy.
- possibly synchronized/high-frequency oscillatory ventilation.
- avoidance of fluid overload.
- closure of patent ductus arteriosus.
- vitamin A (given in some centers).

Question

What is the controversy about corticosteroid therapy?

Antenatal corticosteroids (betamethasone) reduce the severity of lung disease and mortality of VLBW (very low birthweight) infants.

However, when dexamethasone was given to VLBW infants in the first few days of life, it was associated with increased risk of gastrointestinal hemorrhage and bowel perforation.

In infants still requiring oxygen at several weeks of age, a course of dexamethasone sometimes dramatically reduces the oxygen requirement and may allow weaning from mechanical ventilation. However, it is associated with serious side effects:
- short term – high blood pressure, hyperglycemia, increased risk of sepsis
- longer term – Cushingoid facies, hypertrophic cardiomyopathy, catabolic state resulting in osteopenia and failure of growth in length and head circumference, and an increased risk of cerebral palsy.

The optimal dose and length of therapy has not been determined. As a result of the increased incidence of cerebral palsy and other side-effects, it is now used only sparingly and after informing parents of the potential risks. The decline in the use of postnatal corticosteroid therapy is shown in Fig. 25.1.

Inhaled corticosteroids may reduce the need for systemic corticosteroids.

Survival in developed countries of very low birthweight (VLBW) infants has increased dramatically, with the limits of viability now at 23–26 weeks' gestation (Fig. 37.1). However, this increased survival has been achieved at the expense of high rates of neurodisability. Comparing the 1990s with the 1980s, for every 1000 infants below 1 kg in birth weight, an additional eight normal and 11 impaired infants survived.

The development of VLBW infants will be monitored in a follow-up program (see Chapter 69) or in the community. Data on neurodevelopmental outcome should be collected. These can then be compared with data from other units, but such comparisons may be misleading, as the unit's data will be affected by:

• obstetric and resuscitation policies at very early gestations, e.g. infants at 23 weeks may not be resuscitated in one unit but aggressively resuscitated in another unit
• the referral pattern for transfers from other units
• the demography of the mothers attending the maternal unit
• the small sample size of one individual unit, with wide variations from year to year.

The most meaningful outcome data are regional or national, provided the data collection is standardized and complete. A follow-up rate greater than 90% is desirable for all cohorts.

Growth

At discharge from hospital, over 90% of VLBW infants are below the 10th centile for weight, length and head circumference. Many show catch-up growth in the first 2–3 years, first of the head circumference, then weight and then length. Energy requirements are increased (Table 37.1) and growth is improved if the infant is in good health. Catch-up growth is often less in infants with intrauterine growth restriction, and is poorer with symmetric than asymmetric growth restriction (see Chapter 6).

Medical complications

These include:
• bronchopulmonary dysplasia (chronic lung disease) – may require additional oxygen therapy for many months
• gastroesophageal reflux – especially with bronchopulmonary dysplasia (chronic lung disease)
• complex nutritional and gastrointestinal disorders – following necrotizing enterocolitis or gastrointestinal surgery
• bronchiolitis from RSV (respiratory syncytial virus) infection (reduced by giving palivizumab, an RSV monoclonal antibody)
• pneumonia/wheezing/asthma often requiring rehospitalization
• inguinal hernias – require surgical repair.

The commonest reasons for rehospitalization are respiratory disorders and surgical repair of inguinal hernias.

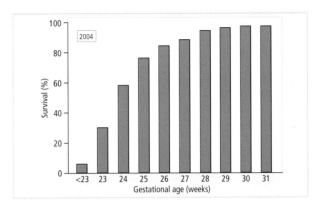

Fig. 37.1 Increase in survival with gestational age. (Vermont–Oxford Network, 2004.)

Table 37.1 Calorie requirements.

Healthy preterm	110–120 kcal/kg/24 hours
Preterm with catch-up growth (kcal/kg/24 hours)	$\dfrac{120 \times \text{ideal weight for length (kg)}}{\text{actual weight (kg)}}$

Neurodisability and behavior problems

VLBW infants are at markedly increased risk of developing cerebral palsy. Its implication for walking and associated disabilities are shown in Table 37.2.

Even if there is no evidence of cerebral palsy, they are more likely than term infants to:
• be poor at fine motor skills, e.g. threading beads
• have poor concentration, with short attention span
• have behavior problems
• have particular difficulty with abstract reasoning, e.g. mathematics
• have difficulty processing several tasks simultaneously.

These become increasingly evident when the individual child is matched against their peers at nursery or school.

They are also at increased risk of hearing impairment, with 1–2% requiring amplification, and of visual impairment, with 1% blind in both eyes.

Table 37.2 Classification of cerebral palsy.

Type	Ambulation (% walking)	Associated disability
Hemiplegia	100	Visual field loss, partial seizures
Diplegia	90	Strabismus, learning and communication disability
Quadriplegia	25	Seizures; hearing, visual and intellectual impairment

School age

Outcomes at 7 years of age of a regional cohort of infants with birth-weight less than 750 g born betwen 1977–79, are compared with those with birth weight 750–1499 g and term infants in Figs 37.2 to 37.4. They show that VLBW infants, especially those <750 g, are at markedly increased risk of:
- impaired growth – they are short and thin
- major impairment – cerebral palsy, and of vision and hearing
- behavioral problems
- impaired cognitive function, often needing special educational placement.

Adulthood

Outcomes of the same cohort of VLBW infants at 20 years of age, compared with term infants, showed that:
- fewer had graduated from high school (74% vs 83%)
- fewer men (30% vs 53%) but not women were enrolled in post-secondary study
- they had a lower mean IQ (87 vs 92) and lower academic achievements
- they had a higher rate of neurosensory impairment (10% vs <1%)
- they had less alcohol and drug use and lower pregnancy rate.

(Data from Hack M *et al.*, Outcomes in young adulthood for very-low-birthweight infants. *NEJM* 2002: **346**: 149–157.)

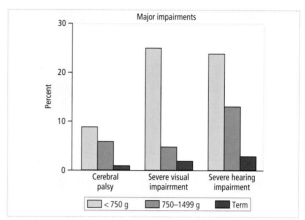

Fig. 37.3 Increased incidence of cerebral palsy, severe visual and hearing impairment in infants with birthweight below 750 g and 750–1499 g compared with term infants. (Adapted from Hack M *et al.*, School-age outcomes in children with birth weights under 750 g. *NEJM* 1994; **331**: 753–759.)

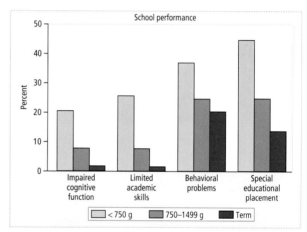

Fig. 37.4 Increased incidence of impaired cognitive function, academic skills, behavioral problems and special education placement in infants with birthweight below 750 g and 750–1499 g compared with term infants. (Adapted from Hack M *et al.*, School-age outcomes in children with birth weights under 750 g. *NEJM* 1994; **331**: 753–759.)

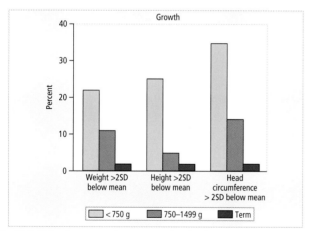

Fig. 37.2 School age growth outcomes showing increased incidence of weight, height and head circumference more than 2 SD below the mean for infants with birthweight below 750 g and 750–1499 g compared with term infants. (Adapted from Hack M *et al.*, School-age outcomes in children with birth weights under 750 g. *NEJM* 1994; **331**: 753–759.)

Overview

The clinical features of respiratory distress are shown in Fig. 38.1.

Monitoring
- Oxygen saturation (maintain >95%).
- Respiratory rate, heart rate, BP, temperature.
- Arterial blood gases if needing oxygen >30%.

Investigations
- Chest X-ray – confirms respiratory disease, excludes pneumothorax, diaphragmatic hernia, lung malformations.
- Complete blood count, blood cultures, C-reactive protein, consider lumbar puncture.

Management
- Airway and breathing – oxygen/CPAP/mechanical ventilation as required.
- Circulatory support if necessary.
- Intravenous fluids or frequent nasogastric feeds.
- Intravenous antibiotics – broad-spectrum coverage.

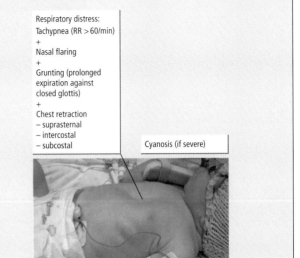

Respiratory distress:
Tachypnea (RR > 60/min)
+
Nasal flaring
+
Grunting (prolonged expiration against closed glottis)
+
Chest retraction
– suprasternal
– intercostal
– subcostal

Cyanosis (if severe)

Fig. 38.1 Clinical features of respiratory distress.

Causes (Fig. 38.2)

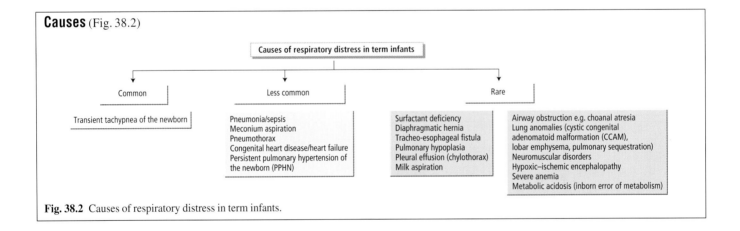

Causes of respiratory distress in term infants

Common

Less common

Rare

Transient tachypnea of the newborn

Pneumonia/sepsis
Meconium aspiration
Pneumothorax
Congenital heart disease/heart failure
Persistent pulmonary hypertension of the newborn (PPHN)

Surfactant deficiency
Diaphragmatic hernia
Tracheo-esophageal fistula
Pulmonary hypoplasia
Pleural effusion (chylothorax)
Milk aspiration

Airway obstruction e.g. choanal atresia
Lung anomalies (cystic congenital adenomatoid malformation (CCAM), lobar emphysema, pulmonary sequestration)
Neuromuscular disorders
Hypoxic–ischemic encephalopathy
Severe anemia
Metabolic acidosis (inborn error of metabolism)

Fig. 38.2 Causes of respiratory distress in term infants.

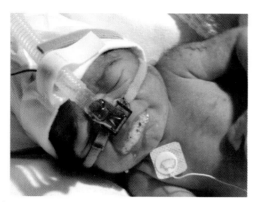

Fig. 38.3 Lung liquid in the mouth of a newborn term infant with transient tachypnea of the newborn requiring nasal CPAP.

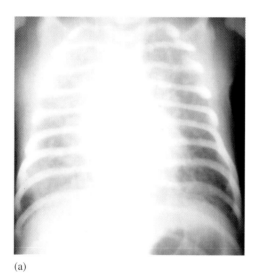

(a)

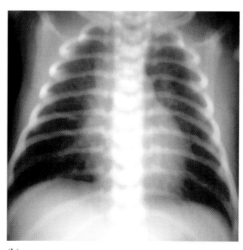

(b)

Fig. 38.4 Chest X-ray in transient tachypnea of the newborn showing fluid in the horizontal fissure and some streaky infiltrates with hyperinflation and perihilar haziness (a). Some hours later, the perihilar haziness has cleared, but there is still fluid in the horizontal fissure and hyperinflation (b).

Common causes

Transient tachypnea of the newborn (TTNB)

This is by far the most common cause of respiratory distress in term infants. Caused by delay in the absorption of lung liquid (Figs 38.3 and 38.4), especially following elective cesarean section. Usually settles within first day or two of life, but may have mild oxygen requirement and take several days to resolve.

Less common causes

Pneumonia

- Risk factors – prolonged rupture of the membranes (PROM), maternal fever, chorioamnionitis, preterm.
- All infants with respiratory distress should be started on broad-spectrum antibiotics until the results of the blood culture, C-reactive protein (CRP), complete blood count (CBC), lumbar puncture (if performed) are known.
- Group B streptococcus is the most common cause.

Meconium aspiration

The proportion of infants who pass meconium at birth increases with gestational age, affecting 20–25% at 42 weeks. Asphyxiated infants may start gasping and aspirate meconium before delivery. At birth infants may inhale thick meconium (see Chapter 12) which results in mechanical obstruction, chemical pneumonitis and inactivation of surfactant (Fig. 38.5). There is a high incidence of air leak. Surfactant therapy may be beneficial. Mechanical ventilation is often required. Accompanying persistent pulmonary hypertension (PPHN) may require nitric oxide and sometimes ECMO (extracorporeal membrane oxygenation), i.e. cardiopulmonary bypass.

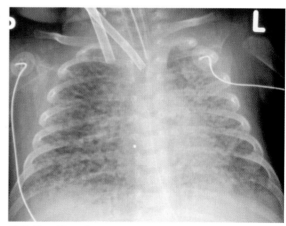

Fig. 38.5 Chest X-ray in meconium aspiration. There is hyperinflation of the lungs, flattened diaphragm and widespread patchy areas of collapse evident in coarse irregular densities with areas of overinflation. There is a tracheal tube and central lines to deliver extracorporeal membrane oxygenation (ECMO).

Pneumothorax (see Chapter 25)

May occur spontaneously or more commonly as a complication of mechanical ventilation or CPAP.

Heart failure (see Chapter 47)

Check for heart murmurs, enlarged liver and that femoral pulses are palpable (reduced in coarctation of the aorta, hypoplastic left heart syndrome).

Persistent pulmonary hypertension of the newborn (PPHN)

Pulmonary hypertension leads to right-to-left shunting of blood (Fig. 38.6):
- across the patent foramen ovale
- across the patent ductus arteriosus

The condition
Usually secondary to:
- perinatal asphyxia
- meconium aspiration
- sepsis
- diaphragmatic hernia.
  Occasionally it is the primary disorder.

Presentation
Cyanosis or difficulty in oxygenation.

Specific investigations
- Chest X ray – shows underlying cause or may be normal or show pulmonary oligemia (diminished vascularity).
- Echocardiography is needed to exclude congenital heart disease.

Management
- Oxygen.
- Optimize mechanical ventilation.
- Circulatory support as required.
- Pulmonary vasodilator – nitric oxide (NO). Sildenafil (Viagra) is being evaluated.
- Consider high-frequency oscillatory ventilation (HFOV) .
- Extracorporeal membrane oxygenation (ECMO) as rescue therapy.

Rare causes
Surfactant deficiency

Rare in term infants. May occur in infants of maternal diabetes or with surfactant protein B deficiency, a rare genetic disorder.

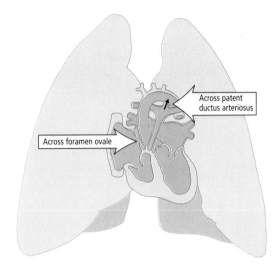

Fig. 38.6 Pulmonary hypertension leads to right-to-left shunting:
- across the patent foramen ovale
- across the patent ductus arteriosus

Diaphragmatic hernia

Main problems
- Pulmonary hypoplasia, as herniated bowel reduces lung development in the fetus.
- Lung compression by the bowel, which increases in size as air enters it.
- Pulmonary hypertension (PPHN) – pulmonary arterioles reduced in number and size, and hypertrophied smooth muscle.
- Other anomalies – present in 15–25%.

Incidence
1 in 4000 births.

Most common site
Left-sided hernia through the posterolateral foramen of the diaphragm (Bochdalek).

Presentation
- **Prenatal** – on ultrasound screening, polyhydramnios. Most identified antenatally.
- **Resuscitation** – failure to respond; deteriorates with bag and mask ventilation.
- **Respiratory distress** – onset may be delayed if underlying lung well developed.

Physical signs
- Respiratory distress.
- Asymmetry of chest.
- Reduced air entry on affected side.
- Apex beat displaced.
- Scaphoid abdomen – from reduced content of bowel.

Diagnosis
X-ray-chest and abdomen (Fig. 38.7).

Management
- Intubate and ventilate from birth. Gentle ventilation, allowing permissive hypercapnea, i.e. $PaCO_2$ >60 mmHg (8 kPa) but maintaining pH >7.25.
- Pass large nasogastric tube and apply suction.
- Stabilize and support circulation.
- Early TPN (total parenteral nutrition).
- Surgical repair – delay until stable and PPHN is resolving.
- Nitric oxide for PPHN.
- Extracorporeal membrane oxygenation (ECMO) – pre- and post-surgery in selected cases.

Mortality
20–30%.

Milk aspiration

Risk of aspiration if infant has cleft palate, neurologic disorder affecting sucking and swallowing or has respiratory distress. Infants with bronchopulmonary dysplasia (chronic lung disease) often have gastroesophageal reflux, which predisposes to aspiration.

Airway obstruction – choanal atresia

The condition
A rare bony obstruction between the nasal cavity and the nasopharynx (Fig. 38.8).

Main problem
Bilateral lesions cause respiratory distress and cyanosis immediately after birth due to airways obstruction as newborn infants are obligatory nose breathers. The airway obstruction is relieved on crying or opening the mouth.

Treatment
- Initial – insert oral airway or tracheal tube.
- Definitive – surgical correction.

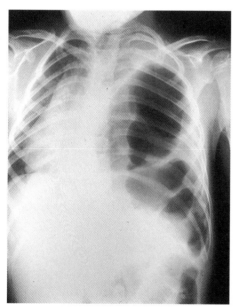

Fig. 38.7 Chest X-ray showing diaphragmatic hernia. There is bowel in the left chest and the heart and trachea are displaced to the right.

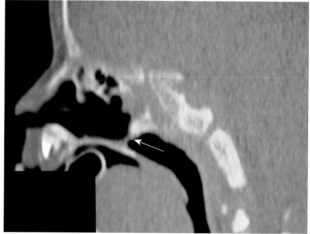

Fig. 38.8 Choanal atresia on MRI scan. There is a bony bar across the posterior nasal space (arrow).

Jaundice occurs in up to 60% of healthy newborn infants. In most it is part of the adaptation to extrauterine life. They become jaundiced because:

• the hemoglobin concentration is high at birth and falls rapidly during the first few days of life
• the lifespan of newborn red blood cells is shorter than that of adult red blood cells
• immaturity of the enzymes in the liver impairs bilirubin conjugation and excretion (Fig. 39.1).

Jaundice is important because:

• a high bilirubin level can cause brain damage (from kernicterus), though this is rare
• there may be an underlying cause which needs to be identified.

Question

What is kernicterus?

Kernicterus is the bilirubin encephalopathy resulting from the deposition of unconjugated bilirubin (Fig. 39.2). The bilirubin is deposited in the basal ganglia and brainstem nuclei. It may result acutely in irritability, lethargy, poor feeding, fever and muscle hypertonicity, resulting in arching of the neck and trunk (called 'opisthotonus'; Fig. 39.3) and seizures, coma and death. Long-term consequences include dental dysplasia with yellow staining of the teeth, high-frequency neurosensory hearing loss, paralysis of upward gaze of the eyes, athetoid cerebral palsy and learning difficulties.

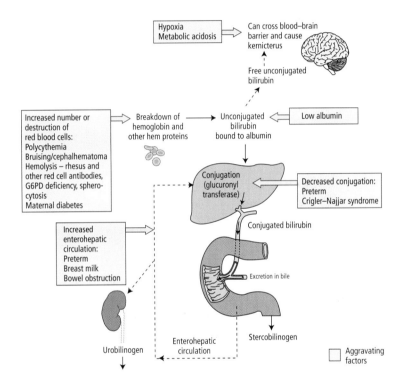

Fig. 39.1 Metabolism of bilirubin. Bilirubin is the product of the metabolism of hemoglobin and other heme proteins. The initial breakdown product is unconjugated bilirubin (indirect bilirubin), which is carried in the blood bound to albumin. When the albumin binding is saturated, free unconjugated bilirubin can cross the blood–brain barrier as it is lipid soluble. Unconjugated bilirubin bound to albumin is conjugated in the liver (direct bilirubin), which is excreted via the biliary tract into the gut. Some bilirubin is reabsorbed from the gut (enterohepatic circulation). Risk factors for jaundice are shown in green.

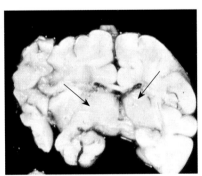

Fig. 39.2 Cross-section of the brain at autopsy showing yellow staining, predominantly in basal ganglia from deposition of unconjugated bilirubin.

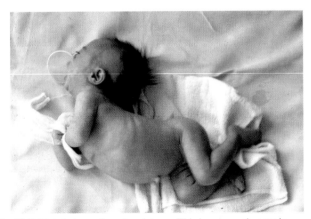

Fig. 39.3 Opisthotonus from kernicterus. This is now rarely seen in developed countries.

Causes

Cause is often categorized according to age of onset (Table 39.1).

<24 hours old

Hemolytic
Jaundice within 24 hours of birth is most likely to be hemolytic. It is potentially dangerous as the bilirubin is predominantly unconjugated (and potentially neurotoxic) and may rise rapidly to very high levels.

RHESUS DISEASE
This is the most severe form of hemolytic disease. Starts *in utero*. At birth, infants may have anemia, hydrops, jaundice and hepatosplenomegaly. Usually identified on antenatal screening tests. Now uncommon because of prophylaxis (see Chapter 5). Antibodies may develop against Duffy and Kell and other blood groups, but are less severe.

ABO INCOMPATIBILITY
- Mother's blood type O.
- Infant's blood type A or B. Maternal IgG anti-hemolysin crosses the placenta and causes hemolysis in the infant.
- Direct antibody test (DAT or Coombs test) is positive (but positive test is poor predictor that the infant will become jaundiced – only 10% need phototherapy).
- Previous sibling may have been affected.
- Less severe than rhesus disease. Onset after birth. Hemolysis with anemia may progress during the first few weeks of life, and this requires follow-up for monitoring for anemia.

G6PD (GLUCOSE-6-PHOSPHATE DEHYDROGENASE) DEFICIENCY
- Affects over 100 million people worldwide.
- May cause severe neonatal jaundice in those with the Mediterranean or Middle or Far Eastern variants and in African Americans.
- Mostly affects males (X-linked recessive disorder); does occur in females but usually less severe. In affected patients, the G6PD level may be normal on laboratory testing if the reticulocyte count is high; the test then needs to be repeated to avoid missing the diagnosis.

- Parents of affected infants should be advised about avoiding:
  - certain medications, i.e. some antimalarials and antibiotics (nalidixic acid, nitrofurantoin and sulfonamides)
  - contact with moth balls (naphthalene)
  - eating fava beans.

HEREDITARY SPHEROCYTOSIS
Uncommon. Positive family history in 75%, as autosomal dominant inheritance. Spherocytes on red cell smear.

Congenital infection
Affected infants may have mild conjugated hyperbilirubinemia. Other stigmata of congenital infection will be present.

24 hours to 2 weeks

Physiologic jaundice
Common. Usually reaches its peak level at 2–5 days of age, then fades.

Breast milk jaundice
Common. Unconjugated bilirubin. Breast-feeding should be continued in spite of it. Will be exacerbated by dehydration from failure to establish breast-feeding or inadequate milk supply.

Continues beyond 2 weeks of age in 15%.

Infection
Always need to consider infection, including urinary tract infection, though it is an uncommon cause of jaundice. Jaundice occurs because of reduced fluid intake, hemolysis, impaired liver function and increased enterohepatic circulation.

Other causes
These include:
- hemolysis – may develop after first 24 hours of life
- bruising, cephalhematoma
- polycythemia
- liver enzyme defects, e.g. Crigler–Najjar syndrome; e.g. rare but causes severe and protracted hyperbilirubinemia
- gastrointestinal obstruction
- metabolic disorders, e.g. galactosemia.

Table 39.1 Causes of jaundice by age of onset.

< 24 hours old	24 hours to 2 weeks old	Older than 3 weeks – prolonged jaundice
Hemolytic	Physiologic	Unconjugated:
Rhesus disease	Breast milk jaundice	Breast milk
ABO incompatibility	Hemolytic	Hypothyroidism
G6PD deficiency	Infection	Conjugated (>20%):
Hereditary spherocytosis	Bruising	Neonatal hepatitis syndrome
Congenital infection	Gastointestinal obstruction	Biliary atresia
	Polycythemia	
	Metabolic disorders	
	Liver enzyme defects	
	Crigler–Najjar syndrome	

Clinical examination and assessment

Jaundice is clinically detectable from skin color on blanching the skin with digital pressure, when bilirubin exceeds 5 mg/dl (85 micromol/L).

It starts on the head, spreads to the abdomen and then to the limbs.

Jaundice may be underestimated clinically and is harder to detect in preterm and Black/dark-skinned infants.

If there is any question about the severity of jaundice, measure the bilirubin level and plot it on a bilirubin chart, according to age in hours (Fig. 39.4).

Check clinically for:
- pallor
- evidence of infection
- bruising, petechiae
- hepatosplenomegaly (in hemolysis)
- weight loss – dehydration.

Investigations

Measurement of bilirubin is indicated if:
- jaundice at less than 24 hours old
- jaundice appears significant on clinical examination.

The total bilirubin is plotted on an hour-specific nonogram to determine the risk of developing significant hyperbilirubinemia (Fig. 39.4).

Further tests, other than total serum bilirubin, that may be required (<3 weeks of age)

- Direct bilirubin.
- Complete blood count, reticulocyte count and smear for red cell morphology.
- Blood type and direct antibody test (DAT or Coombs test).
- G6PD (glucose-6-phosphate dehydrogenase) concentration.
- Serum albumin.
- Urinalysis for reducing substances (for galactosemia).

However, in most infants no cause is identified.

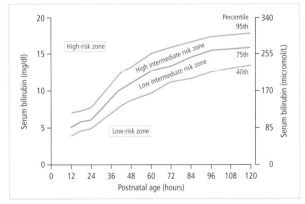

Fig. 39.4 Chart of serum bilirubin by age for infants ≥35 weeks' gestation and ≥2.5 birthweight. This chart can be used to predict risk of developing significant hyperbilirubinemia. (From Bhutani *et al*. Predictive ability of a predischarge hour-specific serum bilirubin for subsequent significant bilirubinemia in healthy term and near term newborns. *Pediatrics* 1999; **103**: 6–14.)

Management

Jaundice may require treatment with phototherapy or exchange transfusion. The need for treatment is ascertained by plotting the bilirubin level on a graph of bilirubin against age in hours. The absolute level and serial measurements showing the rate of rise of bilirubin identify whether treatment is required and whether this is with phototherapy or exchange transfusion (Table 39.2). Different graphs are used for preterm infants, for whom the treatment threshold is lower.

Dehydration associated with failure to establish breast-feeding or inadequate supply of breast milk may require treatment as well as support for the mother to establish breast-feeding.

Sepsis requires investigation and treatment.

Infants with isoimmune hemolytic disease whose bilirubin rises in spite of intensive phototherapy should be given intravenous immunoglobulin.

If an exchange transfusion is being considered, a low serum albumin (high bilirubin:albumin ratio) is an additional risk factor for kernicterus.

Phototherapy

Blue-green light (wavelength 425–475 nm) converts unconjugated bilirubin to harmless isomers. The light is filtered to remove ultraviolet light.

To optimize efficacy requires:
- maximally effective light source
- high level of irradiance (check it regularly)
- correct distance between the light and infant
- widespread skin exposure.

For intensive phototherapy, optimal overhead lights (two if necessary), combined with a fiber optic blanket, are used.

Disadvantages

- Inhibits parental involvement – reluctance to touch, hold and feed their baby (although intermittent phototherapy, within reason, is as effective as continuous).
- Eyes should be covered to protect from bright light.
- Increased evaporative water loss (unless cold light source).
- Unstable body temperature.
- Skin rash.
- Loose stools.
- Bronze baby syndrome if phototherapy given for conjugated bilirubin.

Exchange transfusion

Baby's blood is removed in aliquots (usually twice blood volume, i.e. 2 × 80 ml/kg) and replaced with transfused blood (see Chapter

---

Key points

- If the bilirubin measurement is high on non-invasive testing – check with a laboratory measurement.
- Check that a jaundiced infant is feeding well and is not dehydrated or septic.

Table 39.2 Indications for phototherapy and exchange transfusion in infants ≥ 35 weeks' gestation (Adapted from Management of Hyperbilirubinemia in the Newborn Infant 35 or more weeks of gestation. *Pediatrics* 2004; **114**: 297-316).

Age in hours	Phototherapy			Exchange transfusion		
	Higher risk	Medium risk	Lowher risk	Higher risk	Medium risk	Lower risk
24 hours	>8 mg/dl (137 micromol/L)	>10 mg/dl (171 micromol/L)	>12 mg/dl (205 micromol/L)	>15 mg/dl (257 micromol/L)	>17 mg/dl (291 micromol/L)	>19 mg/dl (325 micromol/L)
48 hours	>11 mg/dl (188 micromol/L)	>13 mg/dl (222 micromol/L)	>15 mg/dl (257 micromol/L)	>17 mg/dl (291 micromol/L)	>19 mg/dl (325 micromol/L)	>22 mg/dl (376 micromol/L)
72 hours	>13 mg/dl (222 micromol/L)	>15 mg/dl (257 micromol/L)	>18 mg/dl (308 micromol/L)	>18 mg/dl (308 micromol/L)	>21 mg/dl (359 micromol/L)	>24 mg/dl (410 micromol/L)
96 hours	>14 mg/dl (239 micromol/L)	>17 mg/dl (291 micromol/L)	>20 mg/dl (342 micromol/L)	>19 mg/dl (325 micromol/L)	>22 mg/dl (376 micromol/L)	>25 mg/dl (428 micromol/L)

Lower risk – ≥38 weeks and well
Medium risk – ≥38 weeks and risk factors or 35–37 weeks and well
Higher risk – 35–37 weeks and risk factors
Risk factors – isoimmune hemolytic disease, G6PD deficiency, asphyxia, significant lethargy, temperature instability, sepsis, acidosis or albumin <3.0 g/dl (30g/L) if measured

74). Now rarely required, except for severe hemolysis. Removes bilirubin and antibodies, and corrects anemia.

Complications include thrombosis, embolus, volume overload or depletion, metabolic abnormalities, infection, coagulation abnormalities. Mortality is probably about 1%.

Discharge

In view of the re-emergence of kernicterus in otherwise healthy infants, particularly at 35-37 weeks' gestation, the American Academy of Pediatrics (2004) recommends predischarge measurement of bilirubin and/or assessment of clinical risk factors for the development of jaundice. It also recommends a follow-up assessment for jaundice depending on their length of stay in the nursery:
- discharge at <24 hours – by 72 hours of life
- discharge at 24–48 hours – by 96 hours
- discharge at 48–72 hours – by 120 hours.

Earlier assessment may be needed if risk factors are present. Parents should also be given written and verbal information about jaundice.

New developments

End-tidal carbon monoxide to detect hemolysis
Carbon monoxide excretion by the lungs is a by-product of the conversion of heme to unconjugated bilirubin. If raised, it indicates increased bilirubin production. If normal, it has a high predictive value in excluding hemolysis.

Heme oxygenase inhibitors
Heme oxygenase converts heme into unconjugated bilirubin. Inhibitors (e.g. tin mesoporphyrin) have been used successfully in infants. Trials are underway.

Question

What is the status of transcutaneous bilirubin measurements?
Technology has improved considerably. It is useful for screening infants into low-, intermediate- and high-risk categories for developing significant hyperbilirubinemia.

Prolonged jaundice

This is jaundice present at more than 3 weeks of age.

It requires further assessment. First, determine if the jaundice is unconjugated or conjugated.
Unconjugated jaundice is common – causes are:
- breast milk jaundice – in 15% of all breast-fed infants, gradually decreases over several weeks
- hypothyroidism – should have been identified on biochemical screening
- infection
- gastrointestinal obstruction – pyloric stenosis
- rare liver enzyme disorders, e.g. Crigler–Najjar syndrome.

Conjugated jaundice (>20% total bilirubin) may be caused by:
- biliary atresia, rare but important to identify as delay in diagnosis adversely affects outcome
- neonatal hepatitis syndrome.

The infant will pass pale stools (no stercobilinogen) and dark urine (from bilirubin).

Detailed investigation of these infants is required.

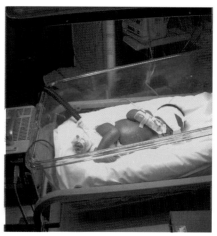

Fig. 39.4 Infant receiving intensive phototherapy with a blue light and fiber optic blanket. The eyes are covered for protection from the blue light. About 6% of all babies are given phototherapy.

This is a common and serious problem in the neonatal period, affecting 1–5/1000 livebirths (Fig. 40.1). The highest incidence is in very low birthweight (VLBW) infants (see Chapter 33). Congenital infections are considered in Chapter 10.

Key point

Infection needs to be considered in all sick newborn infants. If suspected, a blood culture and other investigations should be performed and antibiotics and supportive therapy started immediately as it may progress and disseminate very rapidly.

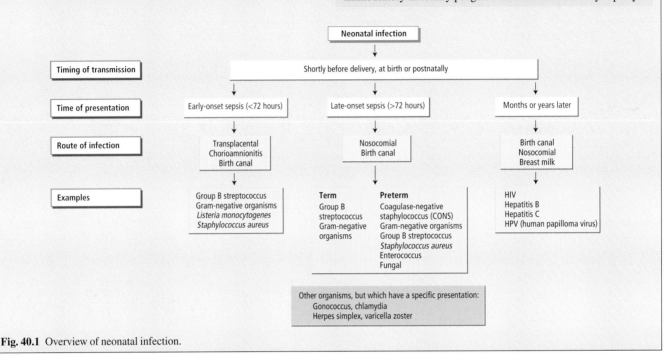

Fig. 40.1 Overview of neonatal infection.

Bacterial sepsis

Newborn infants are particularly susceptible to bacterial sepsis (systemic infection with positive blood or other central culture).

Early-onset sepsis (EOS): <72 hours of birth

Definitions range from 24 hours to 6 days, but most present within 72 hours of birth.

Results from vertical exposure to high bacterial load during birth and few protective antibodies.

Late-onset sepsis: >72 hours after birth

Organisms usually acquired by nosocomial transmission from person to person.

Risk factors

Early-onset infection

- Preterm.
- Prolonged rupture of membranes (>18 hours).
- Maternal fever in labor (>38°C).
- Chorioamnionitis.

- Previous infected infant.

Late-onset infection

- Preterm.
- Indwelling venous or arterial catheters or tracheal tube.
- Prolonged antibiotics.
- Damage to skin from tape, skin probes etc.

Clinical presentation

- Usually non-specific deterioration.
- Apnea and bradycardia.
- Respiratory distress/increased ventilatory requirements.
- Slow feeding/vomiting/abdominal distension.
- Fever/hypothermia/temperature instability.
- Tachycardia/collapse/shock/disseminated intravascular coagulation (DIC).
- Irritability/lethargy/seizures.
- Jaundice.
- Rash.
- Reduced limb movement in bone or joint.
- In meningitis (late signs):
  - tense or bulging fontanelle

– head retraction (opisthotonus).
- On monitoring:
  – hypo/hyperglycemia
  – neutropenia, neutrophilia, thrombocytopenia
  – raised C-reactive protein (CRP).

Investigations

Sepsis work-up:
- complete blood count (CBC), differential, platelets
- C-reactive protein
- blood culture
- urine – microscopy and culture
- cerebrospinal fluid (CSF), if indicated
- chest X-ray, if indicated
- sites of infection – consider needle aspirate or biopsy for gram stain and direct microscopy
- tracheal aspirate if ventilated.

Consider:
- maternal vaginal culture
- placental tissue (*Listeria monocytogenes*)
- rapid antigen screen
- blood gases
- coagulation screen.

Question

When should a lumbar puncture (LP) be performed?
  If blood culture is positive.
  If there are clinical features of meningitis.
  Consider whenever performing sepsis work-up, but delay if infant clinically unstable.
  Skin over LP site needs to be sterile – otherwise may introduce infection.

Interpretation of laboratory investigations

Blood cultures

- Gold standard but may be negative if insufficient volume of blood.
- If central line sepsis suspected, also take blood sample from it.

Blood count

Infection is suggested by:
- neutropenia or neutrophilia
- increased ratio of immature (bands) : total neutrophils
- thrombocytopenia.

C-reactive protein

- Raised in infection; also following meconium aspiration, asphyxia, post-surgery.
- Takes several hours to rise – may be normal initially.

CSF

Meningitis:
- More than 30 white blood cells/mm^3 (30×10^9/L), but more than 20/mm^3 (20×10^9/L) suspicious.
- Protein – term infants >200 mg/dl (>2 g/L).
- Glucose – less than 30% of blood glucose.
- May be able to observe Group B streptococci on Gram-stain without any white cells present.

Treatment

- Supportive care – **A**irway, **B**reathing, **C**irculation. Check blood glucose.
- Treat with antibiotics immediately on suspicion of sepsis, immediately after taking cultures but whilst awaiting results.
- Antibiotic choice depends on local incidence.

Early-onset sepsis
Cover gram-positive and -negative organisms.
  For example:
- penicillin/amoxicillin + aminoglycoside (e.g. gentamicin/tobramycin)

Late-onset sepsis
Need to also cover coagulase-negative staphylococcus and enterococcus.
  For example:
- methicillin/flucloxacillin + gentamicin or cephalosporin/gentamicin + vancomycin

  If central venous catheter in place, remove if unresponsive to antibiotics, persistent positive culture, gram-negative organisms or seriously ill.

Questions

How long should antibiotics be continued?
  If blood cultures are negative and CRP remains normal and clinical signs of sepsis have resolved – stop antibiotics at 48 hours.
  If blood cultures negative but CRP raised – treat as infected.
  If blood cultures are positive – treat until clinical improvement and CRP has returned to normal (5–7 days, longer if gram-negative infection).
  Meningitis – 14 to 21 days.
  Septic arthritis/osteomyelitis – 3 to 6 weeks.

What supportive strategies are being evaluated?
  Giving intravenous immunoglobulin if infected (giving it routinely as prophylaxis in VLBW infants found to be ineffective).
  Giving granulocyte colony stimulating factor (GCSF) – raises white blood count, but efficacy uncertain.
  Exchange transfusion or extracorporeal membrane oxygenation (ECMO).

Group B streptococcal infection

This is the leading cause of bacterial sepsis in term infants.
- Early-onset infection usually presents with respiratory distress and septicemia; more than 90% present in first 24 hours.
- Late-onset infection – higher proportion with meningitis; also causes focal infection in bones or joints.

It is a serious infection, with 4% mortality. Before active prevention, the incidence in the US of early-onset disease was approximately 1.5/1000 live births, late-onset disease 0.35/1000. It was projected that there were about 7600 cases of invasive disease per year, with 300 deaths. By 1999, the infection rate had declined to 0.3–0.6/1000 live births.

Up to 30% of pregnant women have rectal or vaginal carriage of group B streptococcus.

The 2002 CDC (Centers for Disease Control and Prevention) guideline recommends active prevention by culturing all mothers at 35–37 weeks and offering intrapartum prophylactic antibiotics to those who are positive for group B streptococcus (Fig. 41.1). This was shown to be superior to the risk-based screening strategy included in the previous guidelines.

Question

What is the policy in the UK?
In the UK the incidence of early-onset GBS is 0.5/1000 live births and routine culturing of mothers is not recommended (Royal College of Obstetricians and Gynaecologists, 2003). Intrapartum antibiotics:
- should be offered – if previous baby with GBS infection
- should be considered – if preterm labor, prolonged rupture of membranes (PROM) >18 hours, or fever in labor >38°C.

Listeria monocytogenes

- Rare.
- From maternal ingestion of unpasteurized milk, soft cheeses and undercooked poultry.
- Mother develops flu-like symptoms. Fetal infection acquired transplacentally or from birth canal.
- Causes abortion, preterm delivery. Green staining of liquor even though preterm is characteristic.
- Infant – systemic illness or asymptomatic.
- Early-onset infection – usually with pneumonia, septicemia and widespread rash. Mortality 30%.
- Late-onset infection – mostly with meningitis.

Gram-negative infection

- Less common than group B streptococcal infection.
- Presents as early- or late-onset infection.
- Significant morbidity and mortality.

Conjunctivitis

Sticky eyes

Common, 3rd–5th day of life. Clean with sterile water. If troublesome or does not resolve, may be staphylococcal or streptococcal and treat with a topical antibiotic ointment, e.g. neomycin. If persistent, usually due to failure of nasolacrimal duct to open.

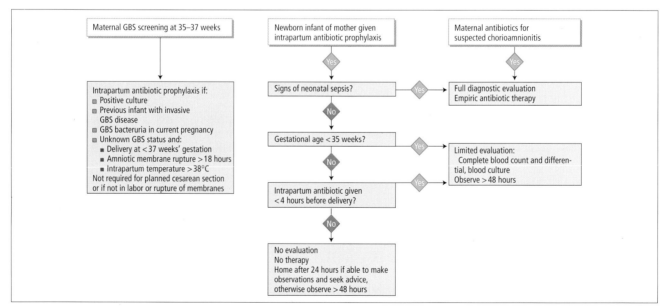

Fig. 41.1 Group B streptococcal (GBS) prophylaxis guidelines in the US. (Based on revised CDC guidelines, 2002.)

Some specific sites of bacterial infection (Fig. 41.2)

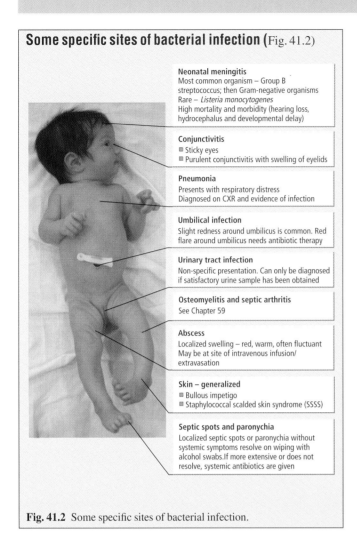

Neonatal meningitis
Most common organism – Group B streptococcus; then Gram-negative organisms
Rare – *Listeria monocytogenes*
High mortality and morbidity (hearing loss, hydrocephalus and developmental delay)

Conjunctivitis
- Sticky eyes
- Purulent conjunctivitis with swelling of eyelids

Pneumonia
Presents with respiratory distress
Diagnosed on CXR and evidence of infection

Umbilical infection
Slight redness around umbilicus is common. Red flare around umbilicus needs antibiotic therapy

Urinary tract infection
Non-specific presentation. Can only be diagnosed if satisfactory urine sample has been obtained

Osteomyelitis and septic arthritis
See Chapter 59

Abscess
Localized swelling – red, warm, often fluctuant
May be at site of intravenous infusion/extravasation

Skin – generalized
- Bullous impetigo
- Staphylococcal scalded skin syndrome (SSSS)

Septic spots and paronychia
Localized septic spots or paronychia without systemic symptoms resolve on wiping with alcohol swabs. If more extensive or does not resolve, systemic antibiotics are given

Fig. 41.2 Some specific sites of bacterial infection.

Purulent conjunctivitis with swelling of eyelids (Fig. 41.3)

If onset within 48 hours of birth, likely to be gonococcal (*ophthalmia neonatorum*). The discharge should be gram-stained and cultured, and systemic treatment started immediately. Where penicillin resistance is troublesome, as in the US and UK, a third-generation cephalosporin is given. The eye is cleaned frequently.

In the US all infants are given eye prophylaxis with erythromycin or tetracycline eye ointment or silver nitrate eye drops. In the UK no prophylaxis is given, but the condition is rare.

Chlamydia trachomatis can cause a similar condition, usually at the end of the first week; may coexist with gonococcal infection. The diagnosis is made with a monoclonal antibody test or culture of the discharge. Treatment is with oral erythromycin. No topical treatment required. These conditions must be treated promptly to avoid damage to the eye. The mother and her partner also need treatment.

Skin

Bullous impetigo

Superficial blisters, readily burst, to leave denuded skin (Fig. 41.4) with crust formation.

Staphylococcus aureus or streptococcal. Give systemic antibiotics to prevent spread. Remove crusts with warm water. Identify and treat source. Usually from nasal colonization.

Staphylococcal scalded skin syndrome (SSSS)

- Rare but serious infection.
- Fever.
- Bullae with shedding of skin leaving raw areas.
- Toxin-mediated.
- Requires systemic antibiotics.
- Congenital Candida may resemble SSSS.

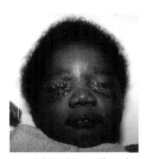

Fig. 41.3 Purulent conjunctivitis with swelling of eyelids at 6 days from *Chlamydia trachomatis*.

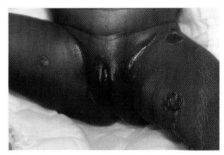

Fig. 41.4 Bullous impetigo. There are superficial blisters; some have been denuded.

Herpes simplex virus (HSV)

Infection in the newborn is rare; the incidence in the US is only 20–50/100 000 live births; in the UK it is 2/100 000 live births. Most (85%) are HSV type II.

Seroconversion rate in pregnancy is 4%.

At any time in pregnancy, 1% of women are excreting HSV.

Risk of vertical transmission

• High (50%) with primary maternal infection, which is symptomatic, with fever, systemic illness and painful genital lesions. Risk of transmission is increased if membranes have ruptured for more than 6 hours or following birth canal interventions, e.g. scalp electrode. However, in 70% of infected neonates maternal infection is undiagnosed.

• Low (<4%) with recurrent maternal infection, which is often asymptomatic or genital lesions are localized.

Potential interventions to reduce transmission of symptomatic primary infection are:

• delivery by cesarean section

• maternal aciclovir (acyclovir) therapy.

Neonatal infection

There are three modes of presentation:

• **Disseminated infection** – presents in first week with pneumonia, hepatic failure, DIC (disseminated intravascular coagulation).

• **Encephalitis** – presents in second week. Lethargy is a prominent clinical feature, as well as stupor, coma and seizures.

• **Localized lesions** – skin, eye or mouth – presents with vesicles at 10–11 days. One-third progress to encephalitis.

Diagnosis

Difficult, as cause of maternal infection often undiagnosed and vesicles present in only 60–80% of disseminated disease or encephalitis.

Rapid diagnosis now with PCR (polymerase chain reaction) of blood, CSF (cerebrospinal fluid), local lesions.

Management of infected infant

• Intensive care support if required.

• High-dose aciclovir (acyclovir) therapy. Giving continued suppressive oral treatment for the first year of life is increasingly undertaken to prevent relapse.

• In spite of treatment, morbidity, mortality and risk of relapse remain high.

Hepatitis B (HBV)

• Highest incidence in the Far East and sub-Saharan Africa (Fig. 42.1). Increased risk with intravenous drug use.

• Screening of all mothers for HBsAg (hepatitis B surface antigen) is universal in the US and UK.

• HBV is transmitted from mother to infant during labor or at birth from ingestion of maternal blood and from breast milk. Also horizontal spread within families during childhood can occur.

• Infants are at high risk if their mother is hepatitis B e-antigen positive (HBeAg positive); the risk is markedly reduced if e-antibodies are present.

• Infants who become carriers are usually asymptomatic during childhood, but 30–50% develop chronic HBV liver disease, which in 10% progresses to cirrhosis. There is also a long-term risk of hepatocellular carcinoma.

Prevention

All infants born to HBsAg-positive mothers should be given HBV vaccination as soon as possible after birth with boosters during infancy. In the US this is part of the standard immunization program; in the UK it is restricted to these high-risk infants.

In the US, HBIG (hepatitis B immunoglobulin) for short-term protection from passive antibody is given within 12 hours of birth to infants of HBsAg-positive mothers; in the UK it is confined to infants of mothers who are HBeAg-positive.

Vaccination protects more than 90% of infants.

Hepatitis C

Vertical transmission is uncommon (<5%) unless there is co-infection with HIV (when it is 10–20%). Risk of transnmission via breast milk is low, so breast-feeding is not contra-indicated. Carriers are at risk of chronic liver disease and hepatocellular carcinoma in later life.

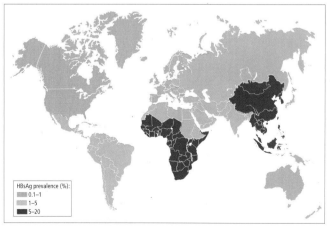

HBsAg prevalence (%):
0.1–1
1–5
5–20

Fig. 42.1 Global overview of prevalence of maternal HbsAg (hepatitis B surface antigen).

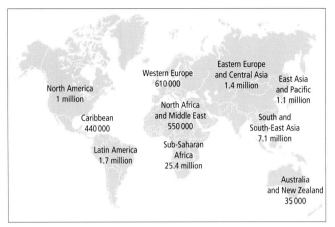

Total: 39 million adults and children
Children < 15 years–2.2 million

Fig. 42.2 Global overview of number of adults and children with HIV infection. (UNAIDS, WHO, 2004.)

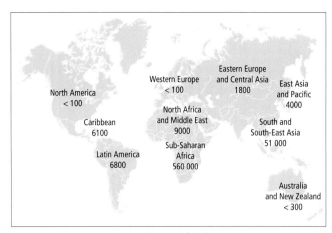

Total: 640 000 infected
AIDS deaths in 2004 – 510 000
Total number of children orphaned (lost one or both parents to AIDS) – 14 million

Fig. 42.3 Estimated number of newly HIV-infected children younger than 15 years during 2004. Most are in sub-Saharan Africa, but there is a substantial number in South and Southeast Asia. (UNAIDS, WHO, 2004.)

HIV infection

The global scale of HIV infection is shown in Fig. 42.2 and how it is affecting children is shown in Fig. 42.3.

Main route of vertical transmission is at birth, but also transplacental and via breast-feeding.

Vertical transmission rate where mothers breast-feed and without any intervention is 25–40%.

Factors which increase transmission

- Advanced maternal disease.
- High plasma viral load.
- Primary infection during pregnancy or breast-feeding.
- Concomitant sexually transmitted infections.
- Rupture of the membranes longer than 4 hours.
- Chorioamnionitis.
- Vaginal delivery.
- Blood exposure/instrumental delivery.

Interventions that reduce transmission

- Anti-retroviral therapy to mother antenatally and postpartum to the infant.
- Treatment of other maternal sexually transmitted infections.
- Elective cesarean section with avoidance of labor and contact with the birth canal.
- Formula feeding instead of breast-feeding (in developing countries, depends on risk and availability of formula milk).

These interventions can reduce transmission rate below 1%.

Diagnosis

Confirmation that the infant is uninfected relies on three negative tests for the viral antigen and/or genome (DNA PCR); antibody tests cannot be used as maternal antibody is detected until 18 months.

Management

Infants should receive cotrimoxazole as prophylaxis against *Pneumocystis carinii* pneumonia (PCP) from 4 weeks of age until negative HIV results are available.

Question

Why are millions of infants throughout the world still acquiring HIV infection?

Reducing transmission to infants requires:

i) identifying that the mother has HIV by testing

ii) giving a short course of antiretroviral therapy to the mother before delivery and to the infant after birth (even a single maternal dose halves the transmission rate)

iii) delivery by cesarean section

iv) ability to safely feed infants of infected mothers by formula instead of breast-feeding.

Unfortunately, this is not possible in many countries.

The ultimate aim must be to avoid maternal infection.

Prolonged symptomatic hypoglycemia can cause neurologic damage. However, during the first few days of life, many breast-fed infants have low blood glucose levels but are asymptomatic; they are able to utilize ketones and other energy substrates. Therefore, the definition of hypoglycemia in the neonatal period has been the source of considerable controversy.

A serum glucose level of less than 45 mg% (<2.6 mmol/liter) during the first days of life is currently accepted as a useful cut-off to establish the diagnosis of hypoglycemia and to initiate active evaluation and treatment. Normal newborn infants produce 4–5 mg/kg/minute of glucose in order to maintain glucose homeostasis.

Risk factors

Antenatal

- Maternal diabetes mellitus – insulin-dependent or gestational (Fig. 43.1).
- Maternal obesity.
- Large or rapid infusions of glucose immediately before delivery.
- Maternal β-adrenergic agonist or antagonist therapy.

Neonatal

- IUGR (intrauterine growth restriction) (Fig. 43.2).
- Large for gestational age.
- Preterm.
- Ill infant – sepsis, etc.
- Iatrogenic – reduced feeds with inadequate intravenous glucose.
- Polycythemia.
- Hypoxic–ischemic encephalopathy (HIE).
- Hypothermia.
- Rhesus disease.

Causes

Risk factors for transient hypoglycemia are listed above. Persistent hypoglycemia is uncommon; its causes are shown in Fig. 43.3.

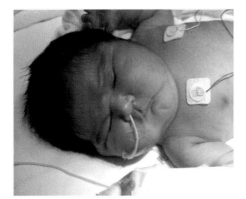

Fig. 43.1 Macrosomic infant of mother with diabetes mellitus. Maternal hyperglycemia causes β-cell hyperplasia of pancreas and hyperinsulinism in the fetus that lasts for up to 48 hours after birth.

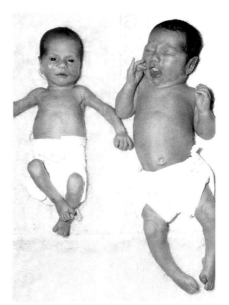

Fig. 43.2 Term twins, the one on the left with IUGR (intrauterine growth restriction). IUGR newborn infants are prone to hypoglycemia.

Clinical features

Most are asymptomatic. Clinical features include:
- jitteriness/irritability/high-pitched cry
- depressed consciousness/lethargy/hypotonia
- apnea
- seizures.

Some abnormal physical signs may assist in identifying the cause (Table 43.1).

Table 43.1 Clinical features associated with specific causes of hypoglycemia.

Clinical feature	Cause
Transient hypoglycemia	
Abnormal growth	Intrauterine growth restriction
	Macrosomia/large for gestational age
Plethora	Polycythemia
Persistent hypoglycemia	
Hepatomegaly with or without splenomegaly	Glycogen storage disease, infection
Hepatomegaly, large tongue, omphalocele, horizontal ear lobe crease	Beckwith–Wiedemann syndrome
Micropenis, hypoplastic optic disc	Panhypopituitarism
	Need to rule out midline brain defects, e.g. septo-optic dysplasia
Lethargy, coma, vomiting, unusual body odor	Hyperammonemia, lactic acidosis, urea cycle disorders or other inborn error of metabolism

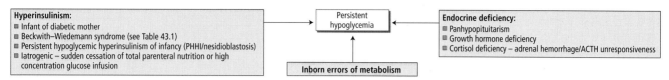

Fig. 43.3 Causes of persistent hypoglycemia.

Monitoring

Infants with risk factors are monitored before feeds until the blood glucose is above 45 mg/dl (>2.6 mmol/liter) on two occasions. It is not necessary to monitor blood glucose levels in appropriately grown term infants establishing breast-feeding. All infants requiring intensive care should have their blood glucose monitored regularly.

Blood glucose determination should be performed at the bedside with a glucometer, which requires only a single drop of blood.

Investigation

These are performed for persistent or symptomatic hypoglycemia.

Blood tests

- Blood glucose concentration – true (laboratory) measurements must be taken.
- Blood insulin concentration.
  If no hyperinsulinism, check:
- pituitary hormones
- for inborn error of metabolism
- acylcarnitine.

Other investigations that may be indicated

- Ultrasound of brain and/or MRI – for structural anomaly.
- Ultrasound adrenals – for adrenal hemorrhage.
- Ophthalmologic examination – for septo-optic dysplasia.

Management

Prevention and treatment of hypoglycemia are shown in Fig. 43.4.

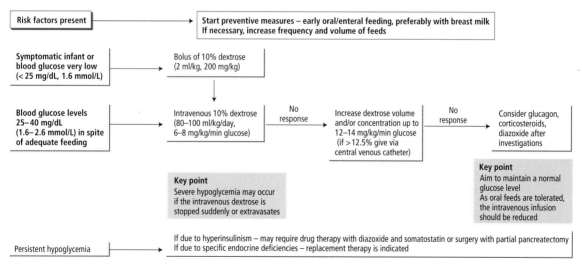

Fig. 43.4 An example of a guideline for the prevention and treatment of hypoglycemia.

There are almost a hundred inborn errors of metabolism that may present in the neonatal period (Table 44.1). They are rare (Table 44.2) but failure or delay in diagnosis can result in irreversible brain damage or death. In the US, tandem mass spectrometry on blood screening spots is used extensively to identify a wide range of metabolic disorders; in the UK screening for inborn errors of metabolism is mostly limited to phenylketonuria and medium-chain acyl CoA dehydrogenase deficiency (MCAD).

Age of presentation

As toxic metabolites are removed by the placenta, most cases present after feeding at several days of age, with acute deterioration of a previously well term infant. Occasionally presents as hydrops fetalis, or as sudden death in the first few days of life. Some present beyond the neonatal period.

Table 44.1 Examples of inborn errors of metabolism that may present in the neonatal period.

Amino acid disorders	Urea cycle – ornithine transcarbamylase
	Maple syrup urine disease (MSUD)
Carbohydrate disorders	Galactosemia
	Glycogen storage disease
Organic acidemias	Propionic acidemia (PA)
	Methyl malonic acidemia (MMA)
Fatty acid oxidation defects	LCAD (long-chain acyl CoA dehydrogenase deficiency)
	MCAD (medium-chain acyl CoA dehydrogenase deficiency)
Energy defects	Lactic acidosis (LA)

Table 44.2 Incidence of some inborn errors of metabolism.

Disorder	Frequency
Phenylketonuria	1 in 10 000
Homocystinuria	1 in 50 000
Galactosemia	1 in 100 000
Maple syrup urine disease	1 in 100 000
If screened with tandem mass spectrometry:	
Amino acid disorders	1 in 4800
Fatty acid oxidation defects	1 in 14 000
Organic acid disorders	1 in 20 000

Investigations when inborn error of metabolism is suspected (Tables 44.3 and 44.4, Fig. 44.1)

Table 44.3 First-line investigations when inborn error of metabolism is suspected.

Investigation	Abnormality	Disorder
Blood gas	Metabolic acidosis	Organic acidemia (MSUD), disorders of carbohydrate metabolism
	Respiratory alkalosis	Urea cycle disorder
Glucose	Hypoglycemia with ketosis	Organic acidemias; glycogen storage
	Hypoglycemia without ketosis	Fatty acid oxidation
Ammonia	Hyperammonenia (Fig. 44.1)	Urea cycle defects, organic acidemia
Lactate	High	Respiratory chain defects, hypoxia
Urea nitrogen (blood urea)	Low	Urea cycle
Electrolytes	Raised anion gap	Lactic acidosis, organic acidemia
Liver transaminases	High	Tyrosinemia, galactosemia
Complete blood count	Neutropenia	Organic acidemias
	Thrombocytopenia	
Coagulation	Prolonged	Liver disease
Urine	Abnormal odor	Organic acidemia
Urine reducing substances	Negative for glucose	Galactosemia
Urine ketones	Positive	Organic acidemias
	Low/negative	Fatty acid oxidation disorders

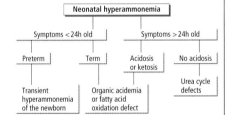

Fig. 44.1 Investigation of hyperammonemia.

Table 44.4 Second-line investigations.

Urine organic acids
Urine amino acids
Plasma uric acid
Plasma amino acids
Plasma carnitine and acylcarnitine
Biotinidase
Galactosemia screening tests
CSF lactate and amino acids
More specialized tests, e.g. enzyme assay on skin fibroblasts or blood cells, DNA mutation analysis, special metabolite assays

When to suspect an inborn error of metabolism

Clinical features

These include:
- Neurologic:
  - poor feeding, vomiting, apnea, irritability, progressive lethargy, seizures, coma.
  - marked hypotonia.
- Acid–base abnormality:
  - persistent, unexplained metabolic acidosis, lactic acidosis or respiratory alkalosis
  - respiratory distress (from metabolic acidosis).
- Hypoglycemia:
  - severe and persistent.
- Acute liver disease:
  - jaundice (conjugated), hepatosplenomegaly.
- Cardiac disease:
  - heart failure, arrhythmias, cardiomyopathy, cardiac arrest.
- Dysmorphic infant.
- Failure to thrive.
- Abnormal body odor.

Suggestive clues

- Positive family history.
- Parental consanguinity.
- Sibling with unexplained severe illness or neonatal death.
- Maternal fatty liver of pregnancy (in fetal fatty acid oxidation defects).
- Sudden onset of symptoms in previously well term infant.
- Progressive deterioration or death despite supportive treatment.

Differential diagnosis

Includes:
- Sepsis – ill with non-specific features.
- Congenital heart disease – heart failure.
- CNS catastrophe – seizures, encephalopathy, infection (herpes simplex virus).
- Gastrointestinal obstruction – vomiting.
- Metabolic derangement – non-specific features.
- Hypoxic–ischemic encephalpathy (HIE) – seizures and encephalopathy.

Management

- Early intervention (Table 44.5) is imperative to prevent neurologic sequelae.
- Dialysis and medical management promote removal of toxic metabolites.
- Keep catabolism to a minimum.
- Empiric treatment may be indicated while awaiting results (Table 44.6). May include special diets, vitamins and carnitine. 5% respond to specific vitamins. Rapid diagnostic testing and clinical history now often allow specific rather than empiric management to be given.

Table 44.5 Immediate management.

Nutrition	Stop feeding, particularly protein and galactose Avoid catabolism – give intravenous glucose
Fluid and circulation	Fluid and circulatory support Correct metabolic acidosis with bicarbonate Correct hypoglycemia
Ventilatory support	Early mechanical ventilation if required
Toxin removal	Hemodialysis or hemodiafiltration
Hyperammonemia	Sodium benzoate, sodium phenylbutyrate and arginine
Insulin	Sometimes used to prevent catabolism
Empiric megavitamin therapy	(See Table 44.6)

Table 44.6 Empiric therapy.

Carnitine
Pyridoxine
Vitamin B_{12}
Biotin
Hydroxycobalamin
Riboflavin
Thiamin
Also coenzyme Q, sodium benzoate, biopterin

Key point

If an inborn error of metabolism is suspected, consult a specialized center for advice on management.

Question

What samples should be obtained if an inborn error of metabolism is suspected in an infant who is preterminal or has died?

Blood spot – on biochemical screening filter paper.

Plasma – heparinized, separated, deep-frozen.

Urine – deep-frozen.

Sample for DNA – blood in EDTA and deep-frozen.

Skin for fibroblast culture – sterile into medium, store at 4–8°C.

Liver for histochemistry or enzymes – snap-frozen.

Muscle and other tissues if indicated – snap-frozen.

Vomiting

This is the forceful return of gastric contents. It is in contrast to regurgitation or possetting, the effortless return of small quantities of milk, which is very common during the first few months of life.

The significance of the vomiting will depend on:
- infant's age
- frequency, amount and characteristics of vomiting, e.g. if projectile
- presence of bile or blood (Figs 45.1 and 45.2)
- abdominal distension
- stool characteristics – delayed passage of meconium or absent transitional stools
- presence of dehydration, weight loss
- evidence of a systemic illness – poor feeding, fever, lethargy.

Causes

Physiologic:
- Gastroesophageal reflux.
- Ingestion of maternal blood.
- Overfeeding.
- Incorrectly positioned nasogastric tube.

Infection:
- Systemic
  - septicemia, urinary tract infection, meningitis.
- Local
  - gastroenteritis.

Mechanical/surgical:
- Intestinal obstruction – see Chapter 46.
- Paralytic ileus – sepsis, electrolyte disturbance.
- Necrotizing enterocolitis – see Chapter 35.

CNS:
- Raised intracranial pressure – cerebral edema, intracranial or subdural bleed, hydrocephalus.
- Kernicterus.

Drugs:
- Side-effects – caffeine, theophylline, antibiotics.
- Withdrawal (abstinence) – heroin, methadone.

Cow's milk protein intolerance

Inborn errors of metabolism (rare)

Endocrine:
- Congenital adrenal hyperplasia (rare).

Diagnostic clues

Bile-stained vomiting (yellow–green)

Causes:
- Intestinal obstruction – distal to ampulla of Vater.

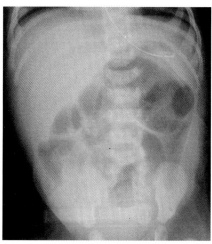

Fig. 45.1 Abdominal X-ray showing distended loops of bowel from meconium ileus. The infant presented with bile-stained vomiting at 30 hours of life.

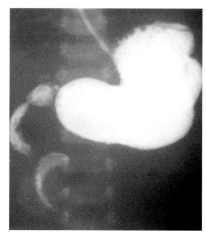

Fig. 45.2 Water-soluble contrast upper gastrointestinal study demonstrating coiled corkscrew appearance of second and third parts of duodenum due to midgut volvulus from malrotation. This infant presented with blood-stained vomiting at 12 hours of age. (Courtesy of Dr Annemarie Jeanes.)

- Necrotizing enterocolitis.
- Incorrectly positioned nasogastric tube.
- Feeding intolerance in very low birthweight infants establishing feeds (common and presence of bile not significant unless there is abdominal distension or features of necrotizing enterocolitis).

Key point

Bile-stained vomiting in term infants should always be regarded as intestinal obstruction until proven otherwise.

Vomiting with abdominal distension

Causes:
- Intestinal obstruction (Fig. 45.3).
- Paralytic ileus – sepsis, electrolyte disturbance.
- Necrotizing enterocolitis.

Investigations

Most infants will require no or limited investigations. Those to be considered are listed in Table 45.1.

Management

Depends upon severity and cause. Intravenous fluids may be required to correct electrolyte disturbances, acid–base imbalance and dehydration.

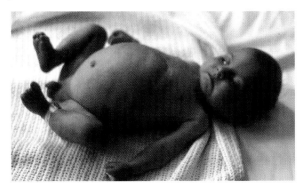

Fig. 45.3 Abdominal distension from Hirschsprung disease.

Gastroesophageal reflux in neonates

Incidence is increased in:
- preterm infants, particularly with bronchopulmonary dysplasia (chronic lung disease) or on caffeine.
- following necrotizing enterocolitis and tracheoesophageal fistula repair.
- infants with neurodevelopmental delay, e.g. following hypoxic–ischemic encephalopathy or hypotonia.

Associated features
- Failure to thrive.
- Irritability, arching of the back from esophagitis.
- Anemia (iron deficiency).
- Aspiration pneumonia.
- Apnea.
- Acute life-threatening events (ALTE).

Investigations
- Usually clinical diagnosis.
- Esophageal pH study, sometimes upper gastrointestinal contrast or endoscopy.

Management
Most do not need treatment. If required, use stepwise approach.
- Reduce interval between feeds, thicken feeds, alginate/antacid (Gaviscon), upright positioning.
- Prokinetic (domperidone).
- H_2 receptor antagonist, e.g. ranitidine; proton pump inhibitors, e.g. omeprazole – reduce gastric acidity.
- Surgery – fundoplication with or without gastrostomy.
  Evidence of efficacy of medication in neonates is limited.

Table 45.1 Vomiting-investigations to consider and their purpose.

Imaging	Blood tests	Urine and stool tests
Plain abdominal X-ray: • intestinal obstruction – distended loops of bowel, bowel perforation • NEC (necrotizing enterocolitis) Ultrasound scans: • cranial for hemorrhage, ventricular dilatation • abdominal for pyloric stenosis Contrast X rays: • malrotation, strictures • site of intestinal obstruction	Electrolytes and acid–base – for imbalance Sepsis work-up to exclude infection Creatinine/blood urea nitrogen – for dehydration and renal function Glucose – for hypoglycemia Calcium, magnesium, phosphorus, liver function tests Coagulation screen – if blood in vomit or sepsis Consider: • 17-hydroxyprogesterone – for congenital adrenal hyperplasia • blood ammonia – for urea cycle abnormalities • drug screen – for drug overdose or withdrawal	Urine – microscopy and culture Stool – for blood Other: APT test of vomit/stool – to differentiate between maternal and fetal blood. Fetal hemoglobin is alkali-resistant (remains pink on addition of sodium hydroxide)

Esophageal atresia

- More than 85% associated with tracheoesophageal fistula (Fig. 45.4).
- 1 in 3500 live births.
- Often associated with other abnormalities, e.g. VACTERL syndrome (**v**ertebral **a**nomalies, **a**nal atresia, **c**ardiac, **t**racheo-**e**sophageal, **r**enal, **l**imb).

Presentation

- Prenatal – polyhydramnios.
- Birth onwards – frothing of oral secretions (Fig. 45.5) with choking and cyanosis.

Investigations

- Unable to pass wide-bore orogastric tube; confirmed on chest X-ray.

Management

- Pass orogastric tube and aspirate pouch to avoid aspiration pneumonia.
- Intravenous fluids for resuscitation and maintenance. Early TPN (total parenteral nutrition).
- Surgical correction is required.

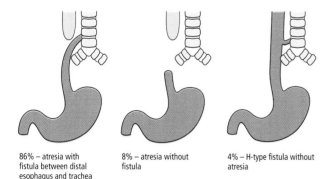

86% – atresia with fistula between distal esophagus and trachea

8% – atresia without fistula

4% – H-type fistula without atresia

Fig. 45.4 Different types of esophageal atresia.

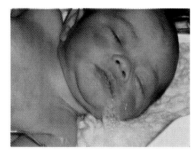

Fig. 45.5 Frothing of oral secretions after birth from esophageal atresia.

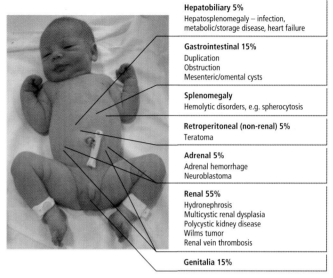

Hepatobiliary 5%
Hepatosplenomegaly – infection, metabolic/storage disease, heart failure

Gastrointestinal 15%
Duplication
Obstruction
Mesenteric/omental cysts

Splenomegaly
Hemolytic disorders, e.g. spherocytosis

Retroperitoneal (non-renal) 5%
Teratoma

Adrenal 5%
Adrenal hemorrhage
Neuroblastoma

Renal 55%
Hydronephrosis
Multicystic renal dysplasia
Polycystic kidney disease
Wilms tumor
Renal vein thrombosis

Genitalia 15%

Fig. 45.6 Abdominal masses and their causes.

Abdominal masses

Often detected *in utero* on ultrasound screening. The causes are shown in Fig. 45.6.

Abdominal wall defects

Omphalocele

Defect in umbilicus with herniation of abdominal contents. The bowel is covered by peritoneum and amnion (Fig. 45.7). Occurs in 1 in 5000 fetuses. Most are diagnosed on prenatal ultrasound screening. In 40% it is associated with trisomy 13 or 18, Beckwith–Wiedemann (see Chapter 43) or other syndromes.

Management
- Pass a large-caliber nasogastric tube at delivery to limit passage of air into the bowel, and nothing by mouth.

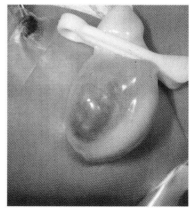

Fig. 45.7 Omphalocele.

- Place infant's lower body into a sterile plastic bag to limit heat and fluid loss and protect the bowel from damage and infection.
- Give intravenous fluids.
- Check for other anomalies, including echocardiography.
- Surgical repair is usually performed on the first day of life. If the defect is large, the viscera may be placed in a Silastic silo, and gradually placed in the abdomen over several days.

Gastroschisis

Defect in anterior abdominal wall, usually to right of umbilicus, with herniation of the bowel (Fig. 45.8). In contrast to omphalocele, there is no protective covering of the bowel and the incidence of associated anomalies is low, other than intestinal atresia from intrauterine volvulus. The condition is usually diagnosed on prenatal ultrasound scanning.

Management
- The infant's lower body is placed into a sterile plastic bag.
- Pass a large-caliber nasogastric tube at delivery to limit passage of air into the bowel.

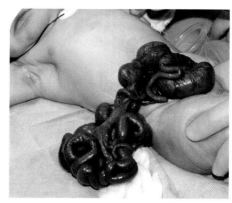

Fig. 45.8 Gastroschisis.

- Give intravenous fluids; colloid may be required to replace fluid losses from the exposed bowel.
- Surgical repair can usually be performed directly.
- Although prolonged parenteral nutrition is usually required to establish feeds, prognosis is good.

Most of the conditions causing gastrointestinal obstructions are serious but their prognosis has improved with advances in medical, anesthetic and surgical care. They are relatively uncommon but are important to recognize because:
• failure or delay in diagnosis may result in electrolyte imbalance, dehydration and shock
• malrotation with midgut volvulus is a surgical emergency.

Causes

These are shown in Fig. 46.1.

Prenatal clues to diagnosis

• **Polyhydramnios** – from obstruction to the passage of amniotic fluid through the gastrointestinal tract.
• **Abnormal ultrasound** – dilated bowel, hyperechoic bowel, ascites, calcified lesions. May be difficult to diagnose.
• **Fetus with trisomy 21 (Down syndrome)** – 30% have associated duodenal atresia.
• **Family history of cystic fibrosis** – associated with meconium ileus.

Delivery room clues to diagnosis

• **Bubbly oral secretions** – esophageal atresia.
• **Peri-umbilical discoloration** – *in utero* bowel perforation.

Clinical presentation

• Vomiting – usually bile (yellow–green stained). Bile is present if the obstruction is distal to ampulla of Vater. Presents within 24–48 hours of birth with high gastrointestinal lesions, may be delayed for several days for lower lesions.
• Feeding intolerance.
• Abdominal distension with visible loops of bowel or peristalsis.
• Erythema/edema of abdominal wall.
• Peritonitis and shock.
• Abdominal mass.
• Failure to pass meconium within 48 hours of birth.
• Blood in stool.

Diagnosis

Abdominal X-ray:
• Bowel obstruction – distended loops of bowel with air-fluid levels, with absence of gas distally.
• Bowel perforation – free air under diaphragm, intrahepatic or around falciform ligament.

Management

• Abdominal decompression with nasal or orogastric tube. In esophageal atresia, need to aspirate pouch to avoid aspiration pneumonia.
• Intravenous fluids for resuscitation and maintenance. Early TPN (total parenteral nutrition).
• Antibiotics preoperatively.
• Evaluate and correct bleeding diathesis.
• Surgical correction for most lesions.
• Evaluate for other anomalies. Karyotype may be necessary.

Some specific conditions
Esophageal atresia

See Chapter 45.

Pyloric stenosis

• **Presentation** – projectile vomiting in a hungry infant at 6–8 weeks of age. Occurs at same age in preterm infants.
• **Examination** – visible peristalsis. A firm, olive-like mass is palpable in right upper abdomen during feeds.
• **Investigation** – Abdominal ultrasound – hypertrophy of pylorus.
• **Management**
  – Correct electrolyte imbalance, hypochloremic hypokalemic alkalosis, before surgery.
  – Surgical correction – incision of muscle (pyloromyotomy).

Duodenal atresia

• **Incidence** – 1 in 7500 births. Check for trisomy 21 and other anomalies.
• **Antenatal** – polyhydramnios, distended fluid-filled stomach on ultrasound.
• **Presentation** – bilious vomiting, upper abdominal distension and feeding intolerance.

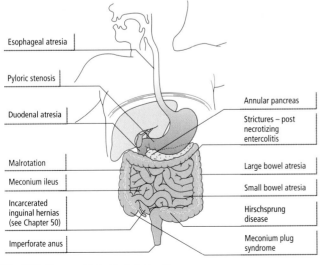

Esophageal atresia

Pyloric stenosis

Duodenal atresia

Malrotation

Meconium ileus

Incarcerated inguinal hernias (see Chapter 50)

Imperforate anus

Annular pancreas

Strictures – post necrotizing enterocolitis

Large bowel atresia

Small bowel atresia

Hirschsprung disease

Meconium plug syndrome

Fig. 46.1 Causes of intestinal obstruction.

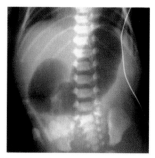

Fig. 46.2 Abdominal X-ray showing double bubble in duodenal atresia.

- **Diagnosis** – double bubble on X-ray (Fig. 46.2). May be accentuated by injecting 20 ml of air through gastric tube.
- **Lesion** – obstruction may be due to atresia, webs, stenosis or fibrous cord.

Malrotation

Failure of the developing bowel to undergo the normal counter-clockwise rotation during the 4th to 10th weeks of embryogenesis. Peritoneal bands (which normally attach the bowel to the central body axis posteriorly and are also known as Ladd bands) compress the duodenum, partially obstructing it. Because the mesentery is not fixed, malrotation predisposes to midgut volvulus (twisting of a loop of bowel around its mesenteric attachment). In addition to intestinal obstruction, compression of the superior mesenteric artery leads to ischemia of the small bowel.

Presentation

Sudden bilious vomiting is malrotation until proven otherwise. With acute volvulus there is also abdominal distension and tenderness followed by shock. Hematemesis (blood-stained vomit) may occur.

Investigation

Doppler ultrasound of mesenteric vessels may be helpful at bedside. Upper gastrointestinal exam (contrast swallow) is diagnostic. The normal position of the duodenal–jejunal junction (Treitz angle) is to the left of the spine. Any other position indicates malrotation. Volvulus classically appears as a spiral corkscrew of the duodenum (see Chapter 45).

Management

Volvulus is a surgical emergency. Ischemia can lead to small bowel infarction requiring bowel resection. Extensive resection of the small bowel carries a poor prognosis.

To relieve the obstruction, the peritoneal bands around the duodenum are divided. Appendectomy is also performed to avoid future confusion if the child has abdominal pain.

Meconium ileus

- Affects 10–15% of patients with cystic fibrosis, whereas 95% of infants with meconium ileus have cystic fibrosis.
- Small bowel obstruction from inspissated, putty-like, sticky meconium.

Presentation

Bilious vomiting, failure to pass meconium, abdominal distension. Edema of abdominal wall suggests peritonitis. Complications include volvulus and perforation.

Investigation and management

- Abdominal X-ray – dilated loops of bowel, air fluid levels and ground glass soap-bubble appearance of meconium.
- Intra-abdominal calcification indicates intrauterine perforation and peritonitis.
- Gastrograffin (water-soluble contrast) enema may wash out the meconium, otherwise surgery is required.
- Check for cystic fibrosis.

Meconium plug syndrome

Presents as a low bowel obstruction similar to Hirschsprung disease.

Hirschsprung disease

- Incidence – 1 in 5000 births.
- Male:female ratio 5:1.
- May be associated with trisomy 21 (Down syndrome).
- Congenital absence of ganglionic cells in the myenteric plexus secondary to defective migration of ganglion cell precursors from neural crest to hind gut. Proximal bowel is normal.
- Accounts for 20–25% of cases of neonatal intestinal obstruction.

Presentation

- Delayed passage of stools – more than 50% do not stool for 48 hours.
- About 50% of affected children present with abdominal distension and vomiting in neonatal period, others when older with constipation.
- May present with enterocolitis – explosive liquid stools, fever and shock.

Investigation

Abdominal X-ray shows distal bowel obstruction – multiple distended loops of bowel with lack of air in the rectum.

Diagnosis

- Rectal suction biopsy for histology.
- Barium enema – excludes other causes of intestinal obstruction and may show transition zone between normal and aganglionic bowel.

Treatment

Surgical repair.

Imperforate anus

- Incidence is 1 in 5000 live births.
- Fistulas to bladder and rectum are common.
- Associated anomalies of genitourinary and gastrointestinal tract are common. Present in 80% of VACTERL association.

Congenital heart disease:
- is the most common group of structural malformations
- affects 6–8 per 1000 livebirths
- accounts for 30% of all congenital abnormalities.

Risk factors

- Chromosomal disorders and syndromes, e.g. trisomy 21 (Down syndrome), microdeletion chromosome 22 abnormalities (for aortic arch abnormalities and Di George sequence), Turner and Noonan syndromes.
- Maternal – diabetes mellitus, teratogenic drugs, e.g. anticonvulsants, fetal alcohol syndrome.
- Congenital infection, e.g. rubella.
- Siblings of affected child – only slight increase in risk.

Presentation

- Antenatal detection on ultrasound screening.
- Detection of a heart murmur.
- Heart failure – respiratory distress/shock.
- Cyanosis.

Antenatal diagnosis

Many lesions are diagnosed antenatally, especially the severe abnormalities detectable on the four-chamber view used for antenatal ultrasound screening (Fig. 47.1), e.g. hypoplastic left heart. Lesions

Classification (Table 47.1)

Table 47.1 Classification of cardiac disorders.

Acyanotic	Cyanotic
Shunts ('holes')	**Transposition of the great arteries** 5%
VSD (ventricular septal defect) 32%	
PDA (patent ductus arteriosus) 12%	**Reduced pulmonary blood flow**
ASD (atrial septal defect) 6%	
Obstruction ('narrowing')	Tetralogy of Fallot 6%
Pulmonary stenosis 8%	Pulmonary atresia
Aortic stenosis 5%	Tricuspid atresia
Coarctation of the aorta 6%	**Total anomalous pulmonary venous drainage (TAPVD)**
Hypoplastic left heart	
Pump failure	
Supraventricular tachycardia (SVT)	
Cardiomyopathy	

In infants with congenital heart disease:
- 10–15% have complex heart disease with multiple lesions
- 10–15% of children with congenital heart disease have abnormalities of other systems

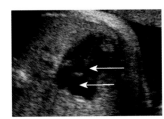

Fig. 47.1 Fetal ultrasound showing atrioventricular septal defect (AVSD).

Key point

About a quarter of infants with congenital heart disease present in the neonatal period and usually have severe lesions.

such as transposition of the great arteries and coarctation of the aorta are difficult to identify.

If risk is increased or an abnormality detected, referral to a perinatal cardiac specialist is indicated. Antenatal detection allows parents to be counseled and postnatal management planned.

Heart murmur

Detected in 1–2% of normal infants on routine examination.

The cause may be:
- **A transient flow murmur** related to circulatory changes following birth. The murmur is soft, systolic, at the left sternal edge or pulmonary area in a well infant whose examination, including four limb blood pressure measurements, is otherwise normal.
- **Pulmonary artery branch stenosis.** The murmur is best heard in the pulmonary area and radiates to the axilla and back. Resolves in a few weeks.
- **Congenital heart disease.** Though uncommon, the most worrying of these are duct-dependent lesions, which may result in circulatory failure or cyanosis when the ductus arteriosus closes. The femoral pulses may be palpable even in coarctation of the aorta shortly after birth as the ductus arteriosus is still patent.

The definitive diagnosis is by echocardiography. A chest X-ray and ECG are of limited value in establishing a diagnosis. Pulse oximetry will establish if the arterial oxygen saturation is normal (>95%). If there are features of an innocent flow murmur, reassess infant within days to check that the murmur has disappeared. The parents need to be informed that they should seek medical assistance should the infant develop symptoms suggestive of heart failure, i.e. slow feeding, breathlessness and sweating. If the murmur persists or has pathologic features or if abnormal clinical features develop, referral to a pediatric cardiologist and echocardiography are indicated.

Key point

The absence of a murmur does not exclude congenital heart disease.

Heart failure

Causes of heart failure and clinical features are shown in Table 47.2 and Fig. 47.2.

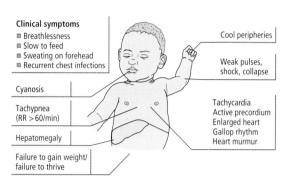

Clinical symptoms
- Breathlessness
- Slow to feed
- Sweating on forehead
- Recurrent chest infections

Cyanosis

Tachypnea (RR > 60/min)

Hepatomegaly

Failure to gain weight/ failure to thrive

Cool peripheries

Weak pulses, shock, collapse

Tachycardia
Active precordium
Enlarged heart
Gallop rhythm
Heart murmur

Fig. 47.2 Clinical features of heart failure.

Table 47.2 Causes of heart failure in the neonatal period.

Left to right shunting (high-output failure)
Patent ductus arteriosus
Atrioventricular septal defect (AVSD)/large ventricular septal defect (VSD)
Left ventricular outflow obstruction
(duct-dependent systemic circulation)
Severe coarctation of the aorta
Critical aortic valve stenosis
Hypoplastic left heart syndrome
Myocarditis/cardiomyopathy
Arrhythmias
Supraventricular tachycardia (SVT)
Non-cardiac
Severe anemia, polycythemia, arteriovenous malformation, e.g. vein of Galen malformation

Selected causes of heart failure

Left to right shunting (high-output failure)

Patent ductus arteriosus in preterm infants
See Chapter 32.

Atrioventricular septal defect (AV canal defect)
- Common (40%) in trisomy 21 (Down syndrome).
- Surgery at 2–4 months.

Large ventricular septal defect
- Only presents at about 1–3 months, when pulmonary vascular resistance is low and left-to-right shunt maximal.
- Surgery if medical therapy fails.

Left ventricular outflow obstruction (low-output heart failure/shock when duct closes)

Severe coarctation of the aorta/interruption of the aortic arch
Key clinical sign is weak or absent femoral pulses. Blood pressure in the arms is markedly higher than in the legs (>20 mmHg). Surgery is required.

Less severe lesions may present as hypertension in adults.

Hypoplastic left heart (Fig. 47.3)
Presents with signs of low cardiac output when ductus arteriosus closes. Pulses are weak at presentation, and there is severe metabolic acidosis. Fatal without treatment – requires a series of palliative operations (Norwood procedure) or heart transplantation.

Hypoplastic left heart

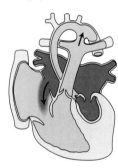

Fig. 47.3 Hypoplastic left heart syndrome.

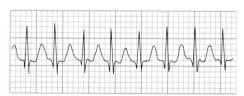

Fig. 47.4 ECG showing supraventricular tachycardia.

Supraventricular tachycardia
- Heart rate 220–300 beats/min (Fig. 47.4).
- Heart is usually structurally normal, but accessory pathway (Wolff–Parkinson–White syndrome) may be present.
- If no response to placing ice pack on face, give the drug adenosine.

Cyanosis

Central cyanosis

- is clinically detectable if there is over 5 g/dl of reduced hemoglobin
- is best detected on tongue/mucous membranes
- in the absence of respiratory distress is usually due to cyanotic congenital heart disease (Table 47.1).

If there is respiratory distress, the cause may be:
- congenital heart disease
- pulmonary disease
- PPHN (persistent pulmonary hypertension of the newborn)
- polycythemia.

Peripheral cyanosis (acrocyanosis)

Hands and feet are blue. Common in infants in the first couple of days of life and in children of any age when cold. The tongue and mucous membranes are pink. It is of no clinical significance in the absence of hypovolemia or shock.

'Traumatic' cyanosis

Cyanosis of the head, often with petechiae from venous congestion, e.g. caused by umbilical cord around baby's neck or face presentation. Tongue is pink. Resolves spontaneously.

Selected causes of cyanotic congenital heart disease

Transposition of the great arteries

In transposition of the great arteries there are two parallel circulations – the aorta arises from the right ventricle and the pulmonary artery from the left ventricle (Fig. 47.5). For survival, mixing of blood between the two circulations must occur, e.g. via the foramen ovale or ductus arteriosus. The less mixing between the circulations, the more severe the cyanosis and the earlier the presentation.

Presentation
Profound cyanosis occurs in the first day or two of life when the duct closes, but may be delayed if there is appreciable mixing of blood from an associated anomaly, e.g. VSD.

Management
This is to promote mixing of the two circulations:
- by maintaining ductal patency with a prostaglandin infusion
- by performing a balloon atrial septostomy to enlarge the foramen ovale (Fig. 47.6).

Surgery will subsequently be required. This is usually the switch operation, in which the pulmonary artery and aorta are switched over. The coronary arteries also have to be transferred to the new aorta, which is technically demanding.

Total anomalous pulmonary venous drainage (TAPVD)

The pulmonary veins, instead of connecting into the left atrium,

Complete transposition of the great arteries

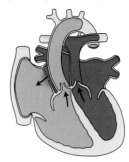

Fig. 47.5 Transposition of the great arteries.

Balloon septostomy

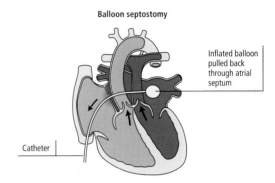

Inflated balloon pulled back through atrial septum

Catheter

Fig. 47.6 Balloon atrial septostomy to enlarge the foramen ovale.

connect into the right side of the circulation, sometimes below the diaphragm.

If the connection is narrow (obstructed) they present with cyanosis, respiratory distress and poor cardiac output. This may be difficult to distinguish from surfactant deficiency. Treatment is surgical.

Investigations

The immediate problem is to distinguish between a respiratory disorder, congenital heart disease (CHD) and persistent pulmonary hypertension of the newborn (PPHN).

Chest X-ray

Helpful to confirm if lung disease is the cause of respiratory distress, bur rarely diagnostic of congenital heart disease as heart size and shape and pulmonary vasculature are difficult to determine in neonatal period. Apparently enlarged heart border may be due to normal thymus.

However, a chest X-ray may show:
- heart enlarged (>60% diameter of thorax), e.g. outflow obstruction from coarctation of the aorta or volume overload, e.g. AVSD (atrioventricular septal defect)
- abnormal shape (e.g. boot shape with tetralogy of Fallot, 'egg on side' with TGA) but often recognized only after the diagnosis has been made

- prominent pulmonary vascular markings (plethoric) from excess blood flow to the lungs, e.g. left to right shunt from patent ductus arteriosus
- reduced pulmonary vascular markings (oligemic) from reduced blood flow to the lungs, e.g. tetralogy of Fallot.

ECG

- Seldom diagnostic; interpretation requires considerable skill.
- Helpful for arrhythmias and as baseline.

Hyperoxia (nitrogen washout) test

May be helpful to distinguish respiratory from cardiac causes (Fig. 47.7).

Interpretation of right radial artery oxygen tension is:
- If PaO_2 >110 mmHg (15 kPa):
  - unlikely to be cyanotic heart disease
  - usually lung disease or PPHN (persistent pulmonary hypertension of the newborn).
- If PaO_2 <110 mmHg (15 kPa):
  - likely to be cyanotic heart disease, but can be severe lung disease or PPHN.

Echocardiography and Doppler

Allow definitive anatomic diagnosis and identification of shunts in most instances. Need good equipment and experienced operator.

Cardiac catheterization

Sometimes required for hemodynamic measurements and increasingly used for interventional procedures, e.g. valvuloplasty.

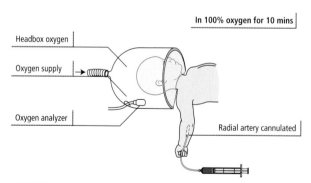

Fig. 47.7 Hyperoxia (nitrogen washout) test to identify cyanotic congenital heart disease.

Management

- Maintain **A**irway, **B**reathing, **C**irculation. Provide ventilatory support if necessary.
- Correct metabolic acidosis, hypoglycemia and hypocalcemia.
- In the first few days of life, give prostaglandin intravenously to keep the ductus arteriosus patent.
- If cyanotic lesion – do not give additional oxygen unless SaO_2 falls below 75%.
- If in heart failure:
  - high-output failure – fluid restriction (acute only), diuretics, ACE inhibitors, e.g. captopril
  - low-output failure/shock – inotropes, volume support; arrhythmias require specific treatment.
- Refer pediatric cardiac center.

Question

Why may giving prostaglandin be life-saving?
By keeping the ductus arteriosus patent when the circulation is duct-dependent. This occurs:
- with obstruction to outflow of the left ventricle, when the systemic circulation is maintained by blood flowing right to left across the patent ductus, e.g. severe coarctation of the aorta (Fig. 47.3)
- with reduced pulmonary blood flow, when the pulmonary circulation is maintained by blood flowing from left to right through the duct, e.g. pulmonary atresia (Fig. 47.8).

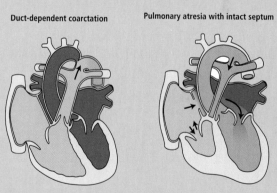

Duct-dependent coarctation   Pulmonary atresia with intact septum

Fig. 47.8 Severe coarctation of the aorta, an example of duct-dependent systemic circulation.

Fig. 47.9 Pulmonary atresia, an example of duct-dependent pulmonary circulation.

Most significant structural abnormalities of the kidneys and urinary tract are now identified antenatally on ultrasound screening. The main exception is vesicoureteral reflux (VUR), which is identified postnatally on specific investigation. Early recognition and treatment may prevent or ameliorate complications such as urinary tract infection, failure to thrive and renal failure. When indicated, it may allow prenatal referral to a tertiary center. The disadvantage is that many minor or transient genitourinary anomalies are identified, resulting in unnecessary concern for the parents and additional investigations for the child.

Embryology

The kidneys and genitourinary tract are embryologically interdependent. If one system is abnormal, look for abnormalities of the other.

Structural abnormalities of the kidneys

Polycystic kidney disease

Autosomal dominant polycystic kidney disease (ADPKD) (Fig. 48.1a)
- Common: 1 in 500 in US.
- Wide spectrum of severity from asymptomatic to renal failure in late adult life. Cysts may not appear until later life.

Autosomal recessive polycystic kidney disease (ARPKD) (Fig. 48.1b)
- Rare: 1 in 10 000–40 000.
- Cysts form in the collecting duct.
- Presents with abdominal masses, hypertension and renal failure.
- Associated with congenital hepatic fibrosis.
- May cause renal failure requiring renal transplant.

Multicystic renal dysplasia (MCD)

- Uncommon: 1 in 4000 live births.
- Renal parenchyma replaced by cysts of various sizes (Fig. 48.2a and b).
- Kidney is functionless, accompanied by atresia of the ureter.

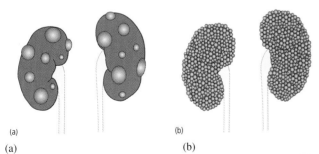

(a)　　　　　　　　　　(b)

(a)　　　　　　　　　　(b)

Fig. 48.1 (a) Autosomal dominant polycystic kidney disease (ADPKD). There are separate cysts of varying size between normal renal parenchyma. (b) Autosomal recessive polycystic kidney disease (ARPKD). There is diffuse bilateral enlargement of the kidneys.

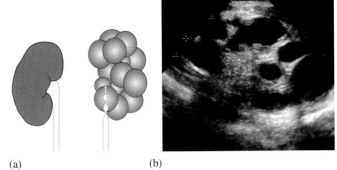

(a)　　　　　　　　　　(b)

Fig. 48.2 (a) Multicystic dysplastic kidney (MDK). The kidney is replaced by cysts of variable size, with atresia of the ureter. (b) Renal ultrasound shows discrete cysts of variable size in multicystic dysplastic kidney (MDK).

- If bilateral, it causes Potter syndrome.
- Kidney may be large and palpable, but more often is small. Contralateral kidney is usually normal, but at increased risk of vesicoureteral reflux.
- Half will have involuted by 2 years. Nephrectomy is only indicated if cysts increase in size or hypertension develops, both of which are rare.

Renal agenesis

- Unilateral agenesis/dysplasia (present in 1 in 1000) is only important if the contralateral kidney is abnormal.
- Bilateral agenesis results in renal failure, causing severe oligohydramnios, as amniotic fluid is mainly derived from fetal urine. The consequence is Potter syndrome, the dominant features of which are from compression because of oligohydramnios (Fig. 48.3). Stillbirth is common; postnatally pulmonary hypoplasia is lethal.

Outflow obstruction

In the fetus with outflow obstruction (Fig. 48.4) there may be:
- hydronephrosis – unilateral or bilateral, with renal parenchyma

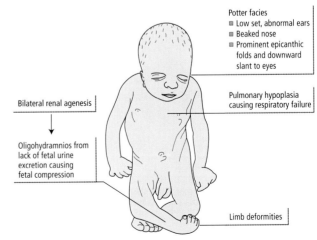

Potter facies
- Low set, abnormal ears
- Beaked nose
- Prominent epicanthic folds and downward slant to eyes

Pulmonary hypoplasia causing respiratory failure

Bilateral renal agenesis

Oligohydramnios from lack of fetal urine excretion causing fetal compression

Limb deformities

Fig. 48.3 Potter syndrome.

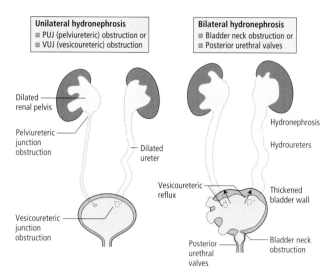

Dilated renal pelvis

Pelviureteric junction obstruction

Dilated ureter

Vesicoureteric junction obstruction

Hydronephrosis

Hydroureters

Vesicoureteric reflux

Thickened bladder wall

Posterior urethral valves

Bladder neck obstruction

Fig. 48.4 Features of unilateral and bilateral outflow obstruction.

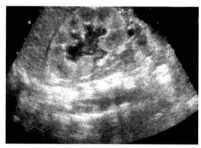

Fig. 48.5 Ultrasound showing unilateral hydronephrosis. As a measure of its severity, the anteroposterior renal pelvis diameter is measured. (Courtesy of Dr Annemarie Jeanes.)

that may be normal or malformed or dysplastic
- dilatation of the ureters and/or bladder
- reduced or absent amniotic fluid volume.

Unilateral hydronephrosis
- Hydronephrosis is dilatation of the proximal collecting system (Fig. 48.5).

- It is the commonest abnormality diagnosed antenatally, and accounts for 50% of all prenatally detected urologic anomalies. It occurs in 1 in 500–700 infants. Most common cause is physiologic hydronephrosis, but others are obstruction at the ureteropelvic or vesicoureteric junction or urinary reflux.
- Management is shown in Fig. 48.6.
- Most but not all resolve spontaneously. Prognosis is dependent on degree of kidney damage resulting from overdistension.
- If the anteposterior diameter does not exceed 15 mm either antenatally or postnatally, intervention is rarely needed.

Bilateral hydronephrosis
Less common than unilateral hydronephrosis but more likely to be serious.

Posterior urethral valves
- Mucosal folds or a membrane obstruct urine flow causing bilateral hydronephrosis, hydroureter and thickened bladder. One third develop end-stage renal failure.
- Incidence is 1 in 5000–8000 live male births.
- Most are diagnosed on prenatal ultrasound, when antenatal intervention may be considered. Options include percutaneous vesicoamniotic shunt placement, bladder aspiration, and drainage of a severely distended kidney. However, outcome after intervention has been disappointing. If there is oligohydramnios, the prognosis is poor.
- Presentation in the infant not diagnosed antenatally includes a palpable, distended bladder, poor urinary flow, renal and pulmonary failure.
- Management postnatally is shown in Fig. 48.6. It is with prophylactic antibiotics, renal and urinary tract ultrasound within 24 hours of birth and VCUG (voiding cystourethrogram, micturating cystourethrogram).
- Treatment – drainage of the urinary tract, initially by urinary catheter, later by ablation of the valves.

Key point

Bilateral hydronephrosis with bladder distension in a boy should be assumed to be posterior urethral valves until proven otherwise.

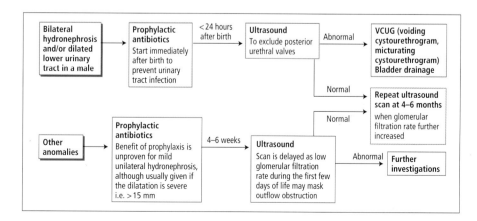

Fig. 48.6 Example of a guideline of the initial management of renal and urinary tract abnormalities detected on antenatal ultrasound.

Renal function in the newborn

Almost all infants void by 24 hours of life. Some key points regarding renal function are listed in Fig. 49.1.

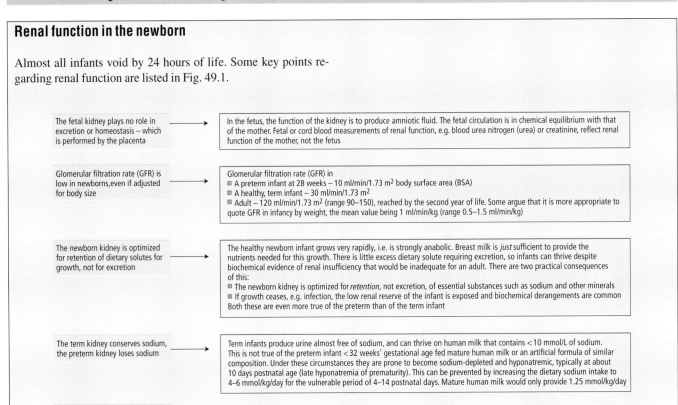

Fig. 49.1 Some key points about renal function in newborn infants.

Acute renal failure

In acute renal failure there is sudden impairment in renal function leading to inability of the kidney to excrete nitrogenous wastes. It is defined as a rise in the plasma creatinine concentration to twice the upper limit of normal, i.e. 1.5 mg/dl (130 mmol/liter) accompanied by a reduction in urine flow rate to <1 ml/kg/hour. However, renal failure can occur without oliguria. It results from a significant fall in glomerular filtration rate with failure of tubular reabsorption of salt and water. It is therefore necessary to monitor the creatinine, blood urea nitrogen (urea) and electrolytes of newborn infants who have been exposed to risk factors for acute renal failure, such as asphyxia, sepsis and aminoglycoside antibiotics (a triad that often goes together), even if they are not oliguric.

Signs of acute renal failure include oliguria, hematuria, proteinuria, hypertension, edema, dehydration, vomiting, lethargy and seizures.

There may be hyperkalemia, acidosis, hyperphosphatemia and hypocalcemia.

In the newborn, mild renal failure is not uncommon in the first few days of life, particularly in preterm infants, and is usually transient.

Prerenal failure, where there is oliguria and nitrogen retention secondary to circulatory inadequacy, responds to volume replacement. In the neonatal period, relatively few cases are due to intrinsic renal damage (acute tubular necrosis), but it does occur in asphyxiated or septic infants. Dialysis is rarely required.

Urinary tract infection (UTI)

Presentation

This is with non-localizing features:
- fever or sometimes low temperature
- poor feeding
- vomiting with or without diarrhea
- jaundice.

  Commoner in boys than in girls – the reverse of older children. Should be suspected in any infant who is non-specifically unwell.

Urine specimens

Methods to collect urine specimens are:
- adhesive bags (high false positive rate)
- urethral catheterization
- suprapubic aspiration.

  In a neonate, if urinary tract infection is suspected, a blood culture and sepsis work-up (with or without lumbar puncture) should be performed as urinary tract infection is usually from hematogenous spread from septicemia (in contrast to older children).

Diagnosis

Depends on the culture any organism of a single strain from a catheter sample or suprapubic aspirate.

Investigations

If culture is positive, ultrasound of the kidneys and urinary tract is performed. A VCUG (voiding cystourethrogram, micturating cystourethrogram) is performed to identify bladder outflow obstruction, e.g. from posterior urethral valves or vesicoureteral reflux (Fig. 49.2). A radionuclide scan (DMSA, dimercaptosuccinic acid or MAG3) is performed several weeks later to identify renal scarring (Fig. 49.3).

Treatment

Antibiotics are started immediately, initially intravenously, whilst awaiting the result of the urine culture (see Chapter 40). Subsequent treatment will depend on the sensitivities of the cultured organism. Treatment should be continued at full dosage until the baby has been well for 2–3 days and a negative follow-up urine culture obtained. Prophylactic antibiotics, e.g. trimethoprim or amoxicillin, should be continued until the result of the VCUG is known.

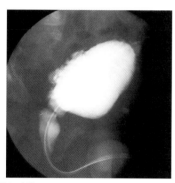

Fig. 49.2 VCUG (voiding cystourethrogram, micturating cystourethrogram) showing trabeculation of the bladder wall, hypertrophy of the bladder and dilated posterior urethra from posterior urethral valves.

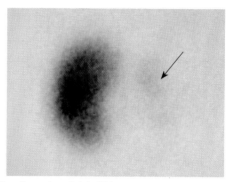

Fig. 49.3 Renal scarring of right kidney (arrow) on DMSA scan on investigation following a urinary tract infection

50 Genital disorders

Features of the normal male genitalia are listed in Table 50.1. Most abnormalities of the male genitalia arise from abnormal embryology (Fig. 50.1).

Inguinal hernia

This is from the processus vaginalis remaining patent. Much more common in males than females and on the right side.

Common in preterm infants, particularly those with bronchopulmonary dysplasia (chronic lung disease) as they have weak muscles and raised intra-abdominal pressure.

Presents as a swelling in the groin or scrotum on crying (Fig. 50.2). It should be repaired promptly to avoid the risk of strangulation in both term and preterm infants, unless the anesthetic risk necessitates delaying the operation.

If the hernia becomes irreducible, the lump is firm and tender. The infant vomits and becomes unwell. It can usually be reduced after sustained gentle compression and opioid analgesia. If possible, surgery is delayed for 24–48 hours to allow the edema to resolve. If reduction is unsuccessful, emergency surgery is required to avoid bowel strangulation and damage to the testis.

Hydrocele

This is fluid around the testis from a processus vaginalis that is wide enough to allow peritoneal fluid to flow down it but too narrow to form an inguinal hernia.

Tense, transilluminates (Fig. 50.3). Often bilateral. Most resolve spontaneously.

Undescended testis

Failure of the testis to descend into the scrotum. Present in 5% of term male infants. Incidence is higher in preterm infants as testicular descent through the inguinal canal only occurs in the third trimester of pregnancy. Testicular descent may continue after birth; by 3 months of age only 1.5% are affected, but few descend thereafter.

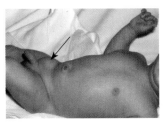

Fig. 50.2 Inguinal hernia in a newborn infant (arrow). (Courtesy of Dr Mike Coren.)

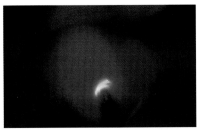

Fig. 50.3 Hydrocele on transillumination. (Courtesy of Dr Mike Coren.)

Table 50.1 Features of normal male genitalia.

Length and diameter – normal size
Meatus – at tip
Testes – palpable in scrotum
Scrotum – rugae

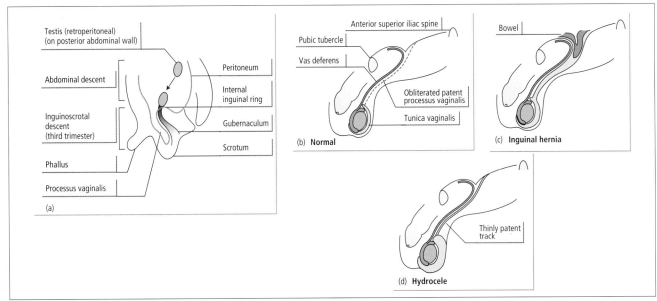

Fig. 50.1 (a) Embryology of testicular descent. The testis migrates from the posterior abdominal wall to the scrotum. It is preceded by a tongue of peritoneum, the processus vaginalis. This is obliterated in the normal infant (b). It remains widely patent in an inguinal hernia (c). With a hydrocele, it is patent but narrow (d).

Examination

With warm hands the contents of the inguinal canal are gently massaged towards the scrotum. If undescended, the testis may be palpable in the groin, but may sometimes be in the abdomen or outside the normal line of descent. If undescended, no testis is palpable in the scrotum, and the overlying scrotum is often poorly formed. A descended testis sometimes subsequently retracts upwards into the inguinal region (retractile testis).

Investigations

For bilateral undescended testes, karyotype may be needed to establish the infant's gender, i.e. male and not a virilized female. The presence of testicular tissue can be confirmed by detecting testosterone production after hormonal stimulation. Sometimes laparoscopy is required to locate the testis.

Management

Surgery to place the testis in the scrotum (orchidopexy) is usually performed during the second year of life because:
• fertility is optimized – the testis needs to be in the scrotum to be below body temperature
• malignancy – there is increased risk, which for a unilateral undescended testis is probably reduced to nearly the same as for a normal testis
• it is cosmetic and avoids psychologic upset.

Torsion of the testis

There is interruption of the blood supply to the testis and epididymis. Occasionally occurs in newborn infants. The testis and surrounding area may be inflamed and the scrotum is black. Must be differentiated from a strangulated hernia and scrotal hematoma. The torsion must be relieved expediently for the testis to remain viable. Doppler ultrasound of testicular blood supply is helpful to determine testicular viability. The testis is seldom viable if torsion is present at birth.

Hypospadias

Common, affecting 1 in 300 boys. In the fetus, the urethra is created by flat tissue folding over from the perineum towards the tip. If this is not completed, the meatal opening may not reach the normal site at the tip of the penis (Fig. 50.4).

In hypospadias there is:
• a ventral urethral meatus – usually on the glans of the penis, but can be on the shaft or perineum (Fig. 50.5)
• a hooded foreskin – from failure to fuse
• chordee – tethering resulting in ventral curvature of the penis, most obvious on erection. This is associated with the more severe forms.

Surgical correction is performed by 2 years of age so that the urethral meatus is at the tip of the penis, erection is straight and the penis looks normal. In most cases of hypospadias affecting only the glans, surgery is not required, except sometimes for cosmetic reasons.

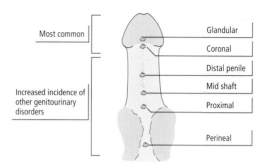

Fig. 50.4 Classification of hypospadias.

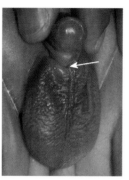

Fig. 50.5 Hypospadias. The urethral meatus is shown by the arrow.

Circumcision

At birth, the foreskin adheres to the surface of the glans penis. These adhesions subsequently separate, allowing the foreskin to become retractile. The foreskin cannot be retracted in 50% of boys at 1 year of age and in 10% at 4 years, but in only 1% by 16 years.

In the US, circumcision is widely performed. In the UK, the main indication is religious, among Jews and Muslims. Its advantages and disadvantages are controversial and emotive.

Advantages are:
• Hygiene – easier to keep clean
• Prevents the possibility of developing phimosis (scarring) or recurrent balanitis (infection) of the foreskin requiring circumcision at a later age
• Slightly reduced incidence of urinary tract infection and sexually acquired HIV infection.

However, it is not a trivial operation, as healing can take up to 10 days. Complications include:
• Pain during and after the operation – adequate analgesia should be provided
• Bleeding
• Infection
• Damage to the glans penis, although this is rare.

Key point

Infants with hypospadias must not be circumcised as the foreskin may be needed at surgery.

51 Disorders of sexual differentiation

In newborn infants, disorders of sexual differentiation present with ambiguous genitalia. There may be:
- virilized female – clitoromegaly, labial fusion
- undervirilized male – micropenis, bilateral undescended testes, poorly developed or bifid scrotum
- true hermaphrodite – both testicular and ovarian tissue present.

They are rare but require prompt evaluation and skilled management to avoid emotional turmoil for parents. Family support and counseling are of utmost importance.

Sexual differentiation

The fetal gonad is initially bipotential (Fig. 51.1).

The testis-determining gene on the Y chromosome (*SRY*) causes differentiation of gonads into testes. Production of testosterone and its metabolite dihydrotestosterone results in the development of male genitalia.

Undervirilization in the male may result from:
- inadequate testosterone secretion from:
  – abnormal testes
  – inability to convert testosterone to dihydrotestosterone (5α-reductase deficiency)
  – abnormalities of the androgen receptor (androgen insensitivity syndrome).
- gonadotrophin insufficiency from:
  – congenital hypopituitarism
  – several syndromes, e.g. Prader–Willi syndrome.

In the absence of the *SRY* gene the gonads become ovaries and the genitalia female.

Virilization is from excessive androgens; the most common cause of this is congenital adrenal hyperplasia.

Hermaphroditism is from chromosomal rearrangement and is rare.

Birth

When a baby is born, the parents immediately want to know if they have a girl or boy.

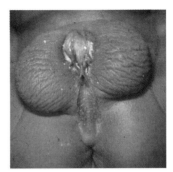

Fig. 51.2 Ambiguous genitalia at birth. Do not guess the gender. (Courtesy of Dr David Clark.)

If the genitalia are ambiguous (Fig. 51.2), it is imperative not to guess but to inform the parents that further evaluation is needed. Birth registration must be delayed until this has been completed.

Investigations

Detailed assessment may include:
- karyotype
- sex and adrenal hormones:
  – blood glucose and electrolytes
  – 17α-hydroxyprogesterone
  – testosterone, dihydrotestosterone and androstenedione
  – hormone (GnRH or HCG) stimulation tests
- ultrasound of internal genitalia and gonads.

Laparoscopic examination and biopsy of internal structures are sometimes required.

Management

Ensure good communication between all health-care professionals so that they do not ascribe a gender to the infant inadvertently.

Most are reared as females, as it is easier to create female external genitalia than a functioning penis, but it is increasingly recognized that this may not necessarily be in the long-term best interest of the

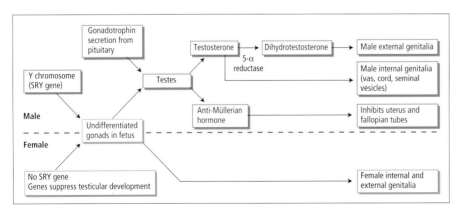

Fig. 51.1 Sexual differentiation in the fetus.

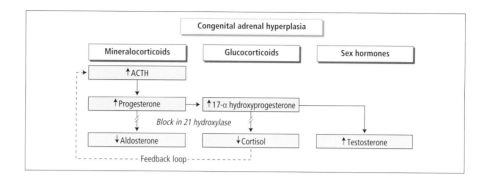

Fig. 51.3 Abnormal adrenal steroid biosynthesis in the commonest form of congenital adrenal hyperplasia (21 hydroxylase deficiency).

child. There is increasing evidence of problems with gender identity, as teenagers and adults, of males reared as females, and evidence of good sexual functioning and satisfaction in males who had a poorly formed penis in the neonatal period. Early referral, expert multidisciplinary assessment and long-term management are required.

Congenital adrenal hyperplasia

- Autosomal recessive condition.
- About 1 in 5000 livebirths.
- Most common cause is a deficiency of an enzyme, 21-hydroxylase, required for cortisol biosynthesis (Fig. 51.3). There is a deficiency in the production of cortisol, aldosterone (salt loss) and an excess of adrenal steroids (virilization).

Presentation

May be with:
- virilization of female external genitalia (Fig. 51.4)
- enlarged penis and pigmented scrotum in male, but rarely recognized
- salt-losing adrenal crisis at 1–3 weeks of age; there is vomiting, weight loss, circulatory collapse which may be fatal; may be accompanied by hypoglycemia
- tall stature, precocious puberty in males.

Diagnosis

Raised blood level of 17α-hydroxyprogesterone.

Management

Short term:
- Salt-losing crisis – requires intravenous saline, dextrose, hydrocortisone.
- Corrective surgery of external genitalia in females.
Long term:
- Glucocorticoids throughout life.

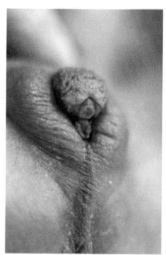

Fig. 51.4 Virilized female from congenital adrenal hyperplasia. There is clitoral hypertrophy and fusion of the labia. (Courtesy of Dr David Clark.)

- Mineralocorticoids if salt loss; infants may need extra oral sodium chloride.
- Monitoring of growth and pubertal development.
- Additional hormone replacement (stress doses) if ill or prior to surgical procedures.
- Further corrective surgery in adolescence to external genitalia in females.
- Psychologic support.

Prenatal testing and screening

Prenatal testing and treatment of affected fetuses are available.

Screening (17α-hydroxyprogesterone concentration) is now performed in most routine biochemical screening programs of newborns in the US but not in the UK.

Anemia

Physiology

In the fetus, the oxygen tension is low. To compensate for this, fetal hemoglobin (HbF) has both a higher concentration and a higher affinity for oxygen than adult hemoglobin (Fig. 52.1).

At birth, the hemoglobin concentration (Hb) is therefore much higher than in an adult. The Hb is also affected by the time of cord clamping at birth and the position of the infant relative to the placenta; if the cord is clamped directly the Hb will be lower than if the infant receives a placental transfusion from delayed clamping and with the baby placed lower than the placenta.

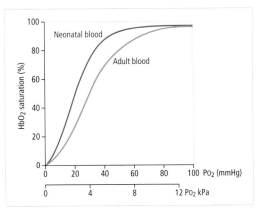

Fig. 52.1 Oxygen dissociation curve showing the higher oxygen affinity of fetal than adult hemoglobin.

Clinical features (Table 52.1)

Table 52.1 Clinical features of anemia.

History	Examination
History – blood loss	Pallor
Family history – anemia, jaundice, splenomegaly	Jaundice from hemolysis
	Apnea and bradycardia
Obstetric history – antepartum hemorrhage	Tachycardia
	Heart murmur – systolic flow murmur
Maternal blood type – Rhesus or other red cell antibodies, potential for ABO incompatibility (mother O, infant A or B)	Respiratory distress, heart failure
	Hepatomegaly and/or splenomegaly, hydrops
	Inadequate weight gain from poor feeding

Management

Blood transfusion

Kept to a minimum because of potential hazards but often required for VLBW (very low birthweight) infants. Erythropoietin is used in some preterm infants to reduce the need for blood transfusions.

Oral iron therapy

Given for anemia or, in preterm infants, to prevent anemia of prematurity. Aim is to not only treat the anemia but also replenish iron stores. Not given if the infant has recently had a blood transfusion.

Oral folic acid

Given as prophylaxis to children with chronic hemolysis. Some neonatal units prescribe it for VLBW infants for the first few months.

Causes and investigation (Fig. 52.2)

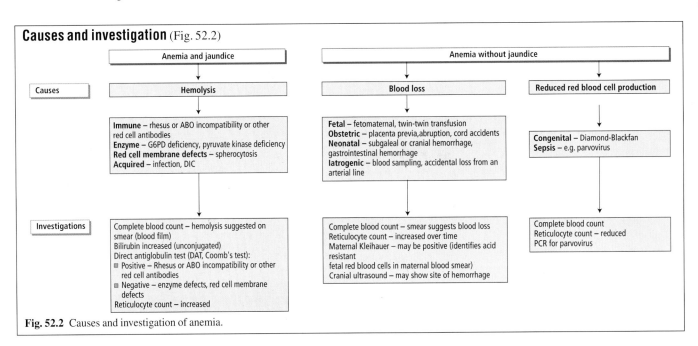

Fig. 52.2 Causes and investigation of anemia.

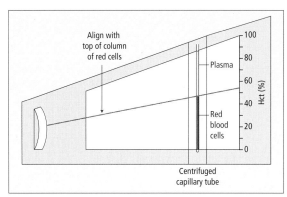

Fig. 52.3 Measurement of hematocrit on a centrifuged blood sample. Centrifuging blood samples is not be permitted in some neonatal units because of health and safety concerns.

Polycythemia

Definition

Usually defined as a venous hematocrit (Hct) above 0.65 (Fig. 52.3). The hematocrit depends on the site of sampling:

- capillary hematocrit > peripheral venous > central venous > arterial.

Potential danger of high hematocrit is hyperviscosity, which causes sludging of red blood cells and formation of microthrombi, leading to vascular occlusion (Fig. 52.4).

Causes

Increased erythropoietin production

- Intrauterine hypoxia – IUGR (intrauterine growth restriction).
- Maternal diabetes.
- Trisomy 21 (Down syndrome).
- High altitude.

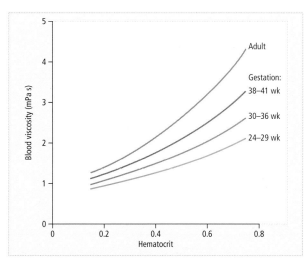

Fig. 52.4 Hematocrit is the main determinant of blood viscosity. Blood viscosity rises exponentially when hematocrit is >0.65.

Increased blood volume

- Placental transfusion from delayed cord clamping.
- Materno-fetal transfusion.
- Twin–twin transfusion.

Clinical features

These are:
- plethora (Fig. 52.5)
- hypoglycemia/hypocalcemia
- irritability, lethargy, seizures
- poor feeding
- hyperbilirubinemia
- respiratory distress
- heart failure
- priapism
- intestinal – necrotizing enterocolitis
- renal – renal vein thrombosis, hematuria, oliguria
- thrombocytopenia.

Treatment and management

There is an increased risk of long-term neurologic impairment in polycythemic infants. However, it is not established that treatment is of benefit as whatever has caused the polycythemia may have also affected the central nervous system. Treatment is to reduce the hematocrit by replacing a proportion of the infant's blood with 0.9% saline. This is done by partial exchange transfusion.

If the venous hematocrit is greater than 0.65 and the infant is symptomatic or the hematocrit is above 0.70 even if asymptomatic – generally agreed that a partial dilutional exchange transfusion should be performed.

If venous hematocrit 0.65–0.70 and asymptomatic – observe and treat only if the infant becomes symptomatic.

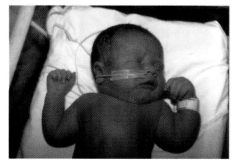

Fig. 52.5 Plethoric term infant. Nasogastric tube is because of poor feeding.

Question

Should one screen for polycythemia?

At-risk infants (intrauterine growth restriction, macrosomia, twins) should have their hematocrit checked. Routine screening of all infants is not recommended because of lack of evidence of benefit of treatment (American Academy of Pediatrics).

Neutrophil disorders

There is a physiologic rise in neutrophils between 12 and 24 hours of life to between 7800 and 15 000 cells/mm³ (between 7.8 and 15 × 10⁹/L), but thereafter the number falls and stabilizes at 1750 cells/mm³ (1.75 × 10⁹/L) at 72 hours (Fig. 53.1).

Neutrophilia

This is an absolute neutrophil count above 15 000–20 000 cells/mm³ (15 – 20 × 10⁹/L).

It is associated with acute bacterial infection, fungal infection and postnatal corticosteroid therapy. When accompanied by a left shift, i.e. increase in immature neutrophils, such as band forms, it is used as a marker for bacterial infection. A normal neutrophil count is helpful in excluding sepsis; the combination of an abnormal absolute neutrophil count and immature:total neutrophil ratio increases the likelihood of infection to about 65%. Serial measurements are more informative than isolated values. However, interpretation of the blood smear requires technical expertise. In the UK it has largely been superseded by measuring CRP (C-reactive protein). Neutrophilia without infection may occur in infants born to mothers with chorioamnionitis.

Neutropenia

This is a neutrophil count of less than 1500 cells/mm³ (1.5 × 10⁹/L). Neutropenia is associated with sepsis, necrotizing enterocolitis, CMV (cytomegalovirus) and other congenital infections, intrauterine growth restriction (IUGR), maternal pre-eclampsia and the chromosome trisomies (13, 18 and 21). Treatment is primarily of the underlying cause. Intravenous immunoglobulin is nonspecific and has not been shown to be beneficial. Recombinant hemopoietic growth factors, in particular recombinant G-CSF (granulocyte colony stimulating factor) and GM-CSF (granulocyte macrophage colony stimulating factor) will increase the neutrophil count, but it is uncertain if they improve outcome. White cell transfusions are rarely effective.

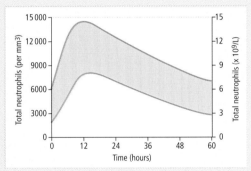

Fig. 53.1 Total neutrophil count, showing the rise with age and the normal range. (From Manroe *et al. J Pediatr* 1979; **95**: 89.)

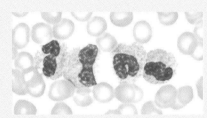

Fig. 53.2 Blood smear showing bands.

Thrombotic disorders (thrombophilia)

A group of disorders characterized by an increased tendency for abnormal clot formation.

Excluding strokes, other thrombotic events have been estimated at 5 per 100 000 births.

Predisposing factors

These are:
- prematurity
- twin–twin transfusion
- cardiac abnormality
- diabetes mellitus
- sepsis
- indwelling catheters
- polycythemia
- asphyxia
- genetic.

Maternal and familial conditions associated with thrombophilia

These include:
- multiple fetal losses
- anticardiolipin antibodies
- SLE (systemic lupus erythematosus)
- maternal diabetes
- placental abruption
- myocardial infarction.

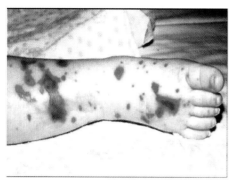

Fig. 53.3 Infant with microthrombi in the skin from protein C deficiency.

Clots and genetics

Gene mutations have been identified for some of the most common thrombotic disorders:
- antithrombin deficiency
- factor V Leiden mutation (APC resistance)
- prothombin gene mutation
- protein C and S deficiency.

Diagnosis

Clinical signs of thrombosis depend on location of the clot, e.g. renal vein thrombosis with abdominal mass, hematuria and hypertension.

Imaging

Depends on site:
- Ultrasound, echocardiography, MRI for diagnosis and follow-up.
- Angiography is the gold standard but may be difficult or not possible to perform or not justified, e.g. for stroke, but MR angiography is now available.

Management

Options include:
- Observe and follow up for increase in clot size and functional compromise.
- Anticoagulation with unfractionated or low molecular weight heparin.
- Clot lysis with fibrinolytic agents (tissue plasminogen activator).
- Surgical thrombectomy.

Strokes

Probably occur in as many as 0.2–1 per 1000 livebirths.

Etiology

May be prenatal, but in most symptomatic infants is perinatal, characteristically in primigravida mother with long or difficult labor and slightly lower Apgar scores and umbilical artery pH compared to normal.

Types
- arterial ischemic stroke (AIS)
- parasagittal or border zone
- cerebral sinovenous thrombosis (CSVT).
  Maternal or fetal risk factors – none in 40–50%.

Clinical presentation

Poor feeding initially, focal signs or seizures on days 1–3, but many are asymptomatic.

Diagnosis
- Cranial ultrasound abnormal in 80–90% infants after day 3 but not always diagnostic.
- MRI for accurate diagnosis and prognosis (Fig. 53.4).

Prognosis

25% of infants with strokes identified in the neonatal period develop a neurologic disability, e.g. hemiplegia later in infancy or childhood.

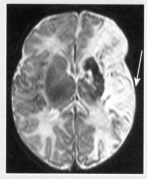

Fig. 53.4 MRI scan showing left cerebral infarct. (Courtesy of Dr Frances Cowan.)

54 Coagulation disorders

In the newborn, abnormal bleeding may be due to:
- a platelet abnormality (number or function)
- abnormal coagulation system
- vascular endothelial damage.

Thrombocytopenia

This is the most common platelet disorder. It is defined as a platelet count of less than 150 000 /mm^3 (150 × 10^9/L). It is usually identified on the complete blood count (CBC), but, if severe, may cause petechiae (Fig. 54.1) or bleeding.

A convenient classification is according to the time of onset (Table 54.1). The most common causes are maternal pre-eclampsia and diabetes mellitus, intrauterine growth restriction and neonatal infection.

Treatment is directed to the underlying cause.

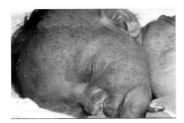

Fig. 54.1 Petechiae from thrombocytopenia in an infant.

Table 54.1 Classification of fetal and neonatal thrombocytopenia (most common causes in bold type).

Time of presentation	Condition
Fetus	**Neonatal alloimmune thrombocytopenia (NAITP)**
	Maternal autoimmune thrombocytopenia (ITP, SLE)
	Congenital infection (CMV, rubella, herpes, syphilis)
	Severe rhesus disease
	Chromosome abnormalities (trisomy 21, 18, 13)
	Inherited (very rare)
Neonatal (<72 h)	**Placental insufficiency (PIH, IUGR, diabetes)**
	Neonatal infection
	Birth asphyxia
	Neonatal alloimmune thrombocytopenia (NAITP)
	Maternal autoimmune thrombocytopenia (ITP, SLE)
	Thrombosis (renal vein, aortic)
	Congenital infection (CMV, rubella, herpes, syphilis)
	Inherited (very rare)
Neonatal (>72 h)	**Late-onset bacterial infection, necrotizing enterocolitis**
	Disseminated intravascular coagulation (DIC)
	Giant hemangioma (Kasabach–Merritt syndrome)

ITP, idiopathic thrombocytopenic purpura; SLE, systemic lupus erythematosus; CMV, cytomegalovirus; PIH, pregnancy-induced hypertension; IUGR, intrauterine growth restriction.
(Adapted from Murray N, *Semin Neonatol* 1999; **4**: 27–40).

For infants who are sick or septic, where production may be compromised, platelet transfusion is given if:
- platelets <30 000/mm^3 (30 × 10^9/L) in term infants
- platelets <50 000/mm^3 (50 × 10^9/L) in preterm infants
- if actively bleeding or before surgery, platelets <100 000/mm^3 (100 × 10^9/L).

These values are a guide.

Abnormal coagulation

Coagulation factors are a group of proteins that upon activation will lead to the formation a fibrin-rich clot or hemostatic plug. These proteins are formed early in gestation in the fetus and do not cross the placenta.

The most common acquired cause of coagulopathy is a combination of coagulation activation and poor liver reserve in a sick or septic infant.

Deficiency of some of the coagulation factors will lead to bleeding disorders (Table 54.2).

Indications for performing clotting studies

These are:
- family history of bleeding disorder
- clinical signs of abnormal bleeding:
  – oozing from venipuncture sites
  – bleeding umbilical cord stump
  – extensive bruising or large cephalhematoma or subgaleal (subaponeurotic) bleed
  – excessive bleeding after circumcision
  – gastrointestinal bleeding.
- septic infant.

Investigations

Coagulation screen consists of:
- PT (prothrombin time) or INR (international normalized ratio of PT)
- APTT (activated partial thromboplastin time)
- TT (thrombin time).

May include:
- fibrinogen
- D-dimers – a measure of fibrin breakdown, useful for diagnosis of disseminated intravascular coagulation (DIC).

Interpretation of abnormal clotting studies (Table 54.3)

The normal values for preterm and term infants are derived locally, as different hospitals use different assays.

The coagulation values in preterm and term neonates differ significantly from older children and adults:
- Prothrombin time tends to be a few seconds longer at birth but will be normal within a week.
- Activated partial thromboplastin time may not reach adult normal

Table 54.2 Bleeding disorders.

Deficiency	Disorder	Comments
Vitamin K	Hemorrhagic disease of newborn	From deficiency of the vitamin K-dependent factors (factors II, VII, IX and X)
		Associated with breast-feeding or severe liver disease in the infant or maternal use of anticonvulsants
Factor VIII	Classic hemophilia A	X-linked inheritance – positive family history in 80%. Mild and moderate forms usually asymptomatic during the newborn period, but after circumcision or other surgery may present with hemorrhage. Severe form may result in life-threatening hemorrhage
Factor IX	Christmas disease – hemophilia B	X-linked inheritance. Similar presentation to hemophilia A
Von Willebrand factor	von Willebrand disease	Most common inherited bleeding disorder
		Autosomal dominant inheritance
		Rarely presents in the newborn period

Question

What is special about taking blood samples for coagulation studies?

Blood sample must be free-flowing. Poor samples cause tissue activation and can give abnormal results, including a normal result in a baby with severe hemophilia.

If the sample is taken from a heparinized line, it may not be possible to interpret the thrombin time. Instead, the fibrinogen and reptilase time must be used as they are unaffected by heparin.

ranges for several months because of low levels of the 'liver' factors (e.g. IX, XI, XII).
• Thrombin time may be slightly prolonged in early life due to the presence of a fetal form of fibrinogen. This is of no clinical significance.

Management of abnormal clotting

If there is active bleeding a correct diagnosis must be established. Vitamin K should be given while results are awaited, and fresh-frozen plasma (FFP) may be given if there is severe bleeding.

If there is disseminated intravascular coagulation (DIC), treat the underlying cause. In the interim, platelets, FFP and cryoprecipitate (only if the fibrinogen level is low) may be indicated. Their need is determined by the coagulation tests, which should be repeated regularly as this is an evolving disorder.

FFP contains all coagulation factors and is suitable for emergencies, but does not contain sufficient of any single factor for severe single factor deficiencies. Replacement by a suitable concentrate is optimal, once a firm diagnosis has been established.

Severe congenital coagulation factor deficiencies – consult pediatric hematologist.

Table 54.3 Interpretation of abnormal clotting studies.

Test	Vitamin K deficiency	DIC	Liver impairment	Hemophilias
Platelets	Normal	Reduced	Normal	Normal
PT	Prolonged	Prolonged	Prolonged	Normal
PTT	Prolonged	Prolonged	Prolonged	Prolonged
TT	Normal	Prolonged	Prolonged	Normal
Fibrinogen	Normal	Reduced	Reduced	Normal

The prothrombin time (PT) may be reported in the form of an INR (international normalized ratio). A normal INR is ≤1.0; an INR >1.1 is equivalent to a prolonged PT. PTT, partial thromboplastin time; TT, thrombin time.

Functions of the skin include:
- mechanical protection
- barrier against microorganisms and toxins
- thermoregulation and fluid balance
- sensory input and tactile communication with the environment.

There are marked differences in the structure and function of the skin of preterm infants, term infants and adults (Table 55.1).

Goals of neonatal skin care

- Avoid traumatic injury during routine care.
- Prevent skin dryness leading to cracking and fissures.
- Minimize exposure to topical agents that are potentially toxic when absorbed (Table 55.2).

Diaper (napkin) dermatitis

Much less of a problem since disposable diapers (nappies).
- Keep skin dry with superabsorbent diapers and frequent changes.
- Treat underlying cause of excessive stooling, such as infectious diarrhea, malabsorption, opiate withdrawal.
- Apply petrolatum to reddened, intact skin to promote healing.
- Apply zinc oxide and pectin paste barriers liberally to excoriated skin to prevent reinjury from fecal enzymes and allow skin to heal.
- Identify candida dermatitis with distinctive pattern of redness on perineum, groin and thighs, and red pustular satellite lesions; apply antifungal ointment or cream. Also, consider oral antifungal treatment.

Add 1% hydrocortisone if unresponsive.

Question

Does the application of an occlusive barrier to the skin of preterm infants reduce transepidermal water loss and desquamation?

This has been demonstrated in a randomized controlled trial using Aquaphor (petrolatum/lanolin). However, it was associated with an increased risk of coagulase-negative staphylococcal infection and is no longer used for this purpose.

Infection

- **Bacterial** – bullous impetigo, staphylococcal scalded skin syndrome (SSSS) (see Chapter 41).
- **Viral** – herpes simplex virus infection (see Chapter 42), CMV and rubella (see Chapter 10).
- **Fungal** – (see Chapter 33).

Vascular skin lesions

Port wine stain (nevus flammeus)

Present at birth in 0.3% of newborns. Most often on the face. Permanent malformation of the capillaries in the dermis. Laser therapy may improve the appearance of disfiguring lesions.

Rare associations:
- trigeminal nerve distribution (Sturge-Weber syndrome) as shown in Fig. 55.1a, intracranial vascular anomaly in 10% (Fig. 55.1b)
- severe limb lesions – bone hypertrophy (Klippel-Trenaunay syndrome).

Table 55.1 Developmental differences between the skin of infants and adults.

Developmental differences	Significance
Stratum corneum	
Term infants and adults: 10–20 layers *<30 weeks of gestation:* 2–4 layers *24 weeks of gestation:* virtually no stratum corneum Also, diminished cohesion between epidermis and dermis as fewer fibrils	*Preterm infants, susceptible to:* • evaporative and transepidermal water loss • transcutaneously transmitted infection and toxicity from topical agents • epidermal stripping with adhesives
Dermis	
Term – only 60% the depth of adults *Preterm* – even thinner dermis, less collagen and fewer fibrils	*Preterm* – excess fluid (edema) accumulates in the dermis, which is prone to injury
Sweating	
Term – limited ability during first few days *Preterm* – unable to sweat before 31 weeks' gestational age in response to heat, although sweat glands are present	Thermal sweating in adults is important to avoid overheating, but newborn infants cannot do this
Emotional sweating of hands and feet – present at term, poorly developed in preterm infants	Emotional sweating to measure response to pain – can be used in term infants, but not in preterm

Table 55.2 Toxicity reported from topical antiseptic use in preterm infants.

Antiseptic	Toxicity
Hexachlorophene	Spongiform encephalopathy
Povidone-iodine	Hypothyroidism, goiter
Alcohol	Hemorrhagic skin necrosis
Chlorhexidine in alcohol	Scalds

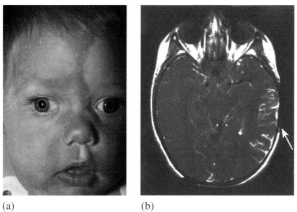

(a)   (b)

Fig. 55.1 (a) Port wine stain with trigeminal distribution (Sturge-Weber syndrome). (b) MRI scan showing intracranial vascular anomaly.

Strawberry nevus (hemangioma)

Not usually present at birth. Appears in first month of life (Fig. 55.2). Preterm infants at increased risk. Increases in size until 8–18 months of age then gradually regresses. May ulcerate. No treatment indicated unless it interferes with vision or the airway, when laser therapy, systemic or inhalational steroids or interferon-alpha may be given.

Congenital melanocytic nevus (CMN) (pigmented nevus)

Small lesions (<1.5 cm) – observe, may remove when older for cosmetic reasons. Small but possible increased risk of malignant melanoma; this contrasts with the much higher risk of giant lesions (>20 cm) (Fig. 55.3), which are treated aggressively. This may be by curettage, when superficial skin containing the pigmentary cells are scraped off within 2 weeks of birth, dermabrasion or surgical excision and skin grafting.

Genetic syndromes

There are a large number of rare conditions (Table 55.3).

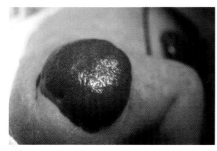

Fig. 55.2 Strawberry nevus. (Courtesy of Dr David Clark.)

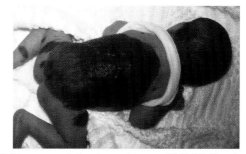

Fig. 55.3 Giant congenital melanocytic nevus (GCMN). Rare but serious condition because of 5–15% risk of malignant melanoma in first decade of life. The lesion may be hairy and satellite lesions are often present. (Courtesy of Prof. Julian Verbov.)

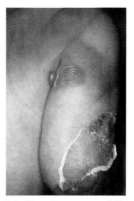

Fig. 55.4 Epidermolysis bullosa. Rare group of disorders. Bullae, or blisters, are caused by trauma or friction to the skin. There are scarring and non-scarring subgroups. (Courtesy of Prof. Julian Verbov.)

Table 55.3 Some skin lesions associated with genetic syndromes.

Skin lesion	Diagnostic group
Unformed skin	Aplasia cutis (absent patch of skin ± bony defect); may be associated with trisomy 13
Thin skin	Dermal hypoplasia, collagen disorders
Blisters/erosions	Bullous disorders, e.g. epidermolysis bullosa (Fig. 55.4)
Thick/scaly skin	Ichthyoses, e.g. collodion infant, or more severe, harlequin fetus
White skin/hair	Pigment deficient disorders, e.g. oculocutaneous albinism, piebaldism, tuberous sclerosis
Palpable brown patches	Syndromes with melanocytic nevi
Flat brown patches	Syndromes with café-au-lait macules, e.g. neurofibromatosis
Deficient hair, nails, sweat	Ectodermal dysplasias. Syndromes with abnormal hair

Seizures (Table 56.1)

Table 56.1 Recognition, causes, investigation and management of seizures.

Recognition	Seizures may present with clonic or tonic involuntary movements of one or more limbs. Often difficult to recognize with certainty, as manifestations are often subtle: • apnea or transient cyanosis, or episodes of oxygen desaturation • lip smacking • transient eye rolling, altered consciousness, floppiness.

Causes	**Cerebral**	**Metabolic**	**Sepsis**	**Drugs**	**Others**
	Hypoxia–ischemia – encephalopathy, birth trauma, vascular Subarachnoid or subdural hemorrhage Parenchymal hemorrhage in preterm infants Congenital malformations of the brain	Hypoglycemia Hypocalcemia Hypomagnesemia Hyponatremia Hypernatremia Hyperammonemia	Septicemia Meningitis or encephalitis	Drug withdrawal: • maternal abuse • following neonatal narcotic therapy Side-effect of drugs	Kernicterus Pyridoxine deficiency Benign

Investigation	**Always performed**	**EEG**	**To be considered**
	Blood glucose (immediate at bedside) Urea and electrolytes Calcium and magnesium Complete blood count Blood cultures Lumbar puncture – protein, glucose, gram stain and culture Blood gases Cranial ultrasound to identify hemorrhage or parietal infarcts or cerebral malformation or abnormalities (may miss subarachnoid hemorrhage)	EEG (Fig. 56.1) or aEEG (amplitude integrated EEG, cerebral function monitoring), which may be combined with video observation – useful to identify seizures (See Chapter 13 for seizures on aEEG) 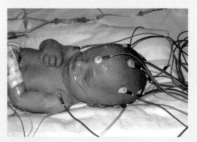 **Fig. 56.1** EEG being performed.	CT/MRI scan of brain to identify malformations, ischemic injury Metabolic screen – plasma for ammonia, amino acids, lactate; urine for amino acids and organic acids Screen for congenital infection Urine for drug toxicology

Management	Airway, Breathing, Circulation. Check for hypoglycemia. Anticonvulsants: • Administer if seizure is prolonged (more than about 5 minutes) or recurs. • No drug shown to be superior to others. Those used include phenobarbital, clonazepam, phenytoin, midazolam, paraldehyde, lidocaine (lignocaine; with ECG monitoring). • Acute seizures often respond poorly. • Use as few anticonvulsants as possible. • Treat the underlying cause, if possible, e.g. sepsis. • If resistant to treatment, consider therapeutic trial of pyridoxine. If caused by acute brain insult, most seizures resolve and anticonvulsant therapy can usually be slowly withdrawn. If maintenance anticonvulsant therapy required – is usually with phenobarbital, clonazepam or sodium valproate.

Cleft lip and palate

Incidence – 1 in 1000 live births.

Inheritance – polygenic, but increased risk if family history.

Varies in severity from a mild unilateral cleft to severe bilateral cleft palate (Fig. 56.2).

It is increasingly diagnosed on antenatal ultrasound scanning. This allows counseling of the parents and family before birth. Showing parents photographs before and after surgery is reassuring as the deformity looks very unsightly.

A specialist multidisciplinary team from a tertiary center is required to provide:
- a key worker, usually a specialist nurse, for advice and to act as advocate for the child and family. Will visit the parents shortly after birth and also gives advice about feeding.
- craniofacial surgeon, orthodontist, speech and language therapist and audiologist.
- surgical repair of the lip, usually at 3 months of age for best long-term results, but some centers perform it immediately after birth. The palate is usually repaired at 6–12 months of age. Further surgery may be required when the child is older.

Long-term complications include middle ear infection and otitis media with effusion, difficulties with speech and orthodontic problems.

There are active self-help groups for parents who provide information and practical help. In the US there is Wide Smiles; in the UK it is called CLAPA, the Cleft Lip and Palate Association.

Choanal atresia

See Chapter 38.

See Chapter 38.

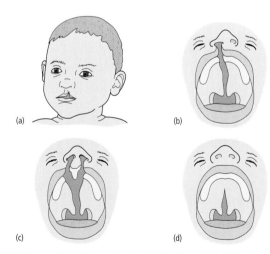

Fig. 56.2 Types of cleft lip and palate. (a) Unilateral cleft lip. (b) Unilateral cleft lip and palate. (c) Bilateral cleft lip and palate. (d) Cleft palate.

Questions

Can babies with a cleft lip and palate breast-feed?

Yes, it is often possible, with expert assistance and encouragement.

What help with feeding can be provided for parents if their infant has a cleft lip and palate?

Special nipples (teats) are available and a dental plate may need to be made to occlude the cleft palate.

Pierre Robin sequence

This comprises (Fig. 56.3):
- micrognathia (small jaw)
- posteriorly displaced tongue
- posterior palatal defect
- increased incidence of other anomalies, especially of the heart.

Most serious complication is respiratory obstruction; may lead to hypoxia and *cor pulmonale* (pulmonary hypertension).

Management

- Avoid obstruction by the tongue:
  - nurse prone
  - may need CPAP (continuous positive airway pressure) via nasopharyngeal tube.
- Micrognathia and airway obstruction improve over the first 2 years.
- Surgery to the posterior palate is usually performed at about 1 year.
- Feeding can be problematic and initially nasogastric feeding may be required.

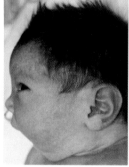

Fig. 56.3 Pierre Robin sequence. (Courtesy of Dr David Clark.)

Neural tube defects

In the embryo, the flat neural plate folds to become the brain and spinal cord. Neural tube defects arise from a deficiency in this process:
- anencephaly – from failure of cranial development of most of the cranium and brain
- spina bifida –from failure of caudal development of the vertebral bodies and spinal cord
- midline defects – from failure of fusion, e.g. of the skull as an encephalocele.

Most are now diagnosed antenatally, by ultrasound or α-fetoprotein measurement in maternal serum.

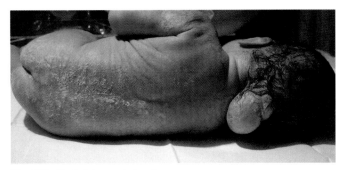

Fig. 57.1 Occipital encephalocele.

Prevalence

There is a combination of environmental and genetic factors. The risk of having a second affected infant is 3–5% and of a third 5–10%. The risk is reduced by maternal folic acid supplementation periconceptually and during early pregnancy.

In the US folic acid has been added to bread and other grain products since 1998 and the birth prevalence has dropped from 38 to 30 per 100 000 live births, a 19% reduction. Other reasons for this are a natural decline and antenatal diagnosis and termination of pregnancy.

In the UK, food is not fortified with folic acid, so folic acid supplementation in low dose is recommended for all women planning a pregnancy, but compliance is poor. High-dose folic acid is given after a previously affected infant. The birth prevalence in the UK is 14 per 100 000 live births.

Anencephaly

The condition is lethal; most are stillborn. There has been considerable debate about the ethics of the use of their organs for donor transplantation. However, the situation rarely arises because few anencephalic infants are now born as most are diagnosed antenatally and parents opt for termination of pregnancy.

Encephalocele

Herniation of sac, which may contain brain, through a midline skull defect. Most are occipital (Fig. 57.1). Developmental impairment is likely if brain tissue is in the sac or there are other cerebral malformations.

Spina bifida

There are several types, of increasing severity:
- spina bifida occulta (Fig. 57.2a)
- meningocele (Fig. 57.2b)
- myelomeningocele (Figs. 57.2c and d).

Spina bifida occulta

If skin lesion is over lower spine there is no neurologic deficit at birth but tethering of the spinal cord may occur during childhood.

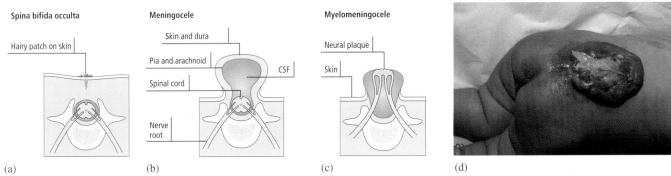

Fig. 57.2 (a) Spina bifida occulta. Defect in the vertebral arch with intact spinal cord. Frequent finding on X-rays – asymptomatic. More extensive lesions indicated by overlying patch of hair or nevus or other skin abnormality. (b) Meningocele. Bony defect with herniation of meninges but not the spinal cord. The lesion is covered with skin. (c) Myelomeningocele. Defect in the lumbar or thoracic spine with herniation of the meningeal sac and spinal cord tissue with leakage of CSF. (d) Photograph of myelomeningocele (myelo = cord; meninges = covering, cele = sac) showing exposed neural tissue and patulous, neuropathic anus.

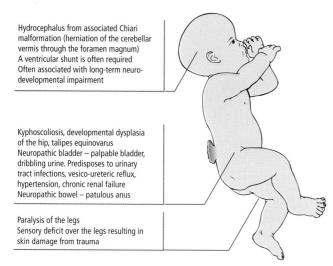

Hydrocephalus from associated Chiari malformation (herniation of the cerebellar vermis through the foramen magnum) A ventricular shunt is often required Often associated with long-term neuro-developmental impairment

Kyphoscoliosis, developmental dysplasia of the hip, talipes equinovarus Neuropathic bladder – palpable bladder, dribbling urine. Predisposes to urinary tract infections, vesico-ureteric reflux, hypertension, chronic renal failure Neuropathic bowel – patulous anus

Paralysis of the legs Sensory deficit over the legs resulting in skin damage from trauma

Fig. 57.3 Complications associated with severe myelomeningocele. These depend on the extent and level of the lesion.

An ultrasound or MRI scan of the spine is indicated and a neurosurgical opinion should be sought.

Meningocele

Prognosis following surgery is usually good.

Myelomeningocele

Wide range of complications (Fig. 57.3). Most lesions are detected antenatally and a management plan made before the baby is born.

Management requires an extensive multidisciplinary team (pediatrics, orthopedics, neurosurgery, urology, child development) and the parents and family.

The back lesion is usually closed immediately after birth to minimize the risk of infection and monitoring performed for hydrocephalus.

Hydrocephalus

This is from an excessive volume of cerebrospinal fluid (CSF). It is usually from blockage of CSF flow or a defect in CSF reabsorption.

Causes

Congenital
- Aqueduct stenosis.
- Chiari malformation.
- Atresia of outflow foramina of fourth ventricle (Dandy–Walker syndrome).
- Congenital infection.

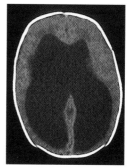

Fig. 57.4 CT scan showing ventricular dilatation in a term infant. (Courtesy of Dr Richard Nicholl.)

Acquired
- Post-intrventricular hemorrhage in preterm infants.
- Post-intracranial infection.
- Post-subdural/subarachnoid hemorrhage.

Clinical features

- Ventricular dilatation on imaging precedes symptoms or signs (Fig. 57.4).
- Increasing head circumference.
- Separation of sutures.
- Vomiting.
- Apnea, abnormal muscle tone, seizures, depressed consciousness.
- Dilatation of head veins.
- Setting-sun sign (eyes deviate downwards).
- Full then bulging fontanel.

Monitoring and treatment

In neonates, hydrocephalus is monitored by serial cranial ultrasound measurements of ventricular size and head circumference.

If severe and progressive or the infant becomes symptomatic, a ventricular shunt is inserted surgically.

Hydrocephalus in preterm infants

This is usually secondary to intraventricular hemorrhage, which may cause obstruction but mainly interferes with CSF reabsorption. The ventricular dilatation may regress, but if it progresses a ventricular shunt will be required. Ventricular shunt insertion in small infants may have to be delayed because of the risk of skin breakdown or if the CSF protein is high, which increases the risk of shunt blockage. If the infant becomes symptomatic but a shunt cannot be inserted, CSF may need to be removed by lumbar or ventricular puncture. A large randomized trial showed no difference in long-term outcome between repeated lumbar/ventricular taps compared with removal of CSF only when symptomatic. Drug treatment with acetazolamide, which reduces CSF production, is not used as it has been shown to be ineffective and carries a risk of electrolyte imbalance. Therapy with fibrinolytic agents is under investigation.

The 'hypotonic infant' describes marked hypotonia or floppiness, i.e. less resistance to passive movement than normal, and is usually accompanied by muscle weakness (Fig. 58.1a, b and c). The cause of the hypotonia is either:
- **central** – central nervous system, or
- **peripheral** – lower motor neuron, neuromuscular junction or muscle disorders.

The level of dysfunction needs to be established.

Transient hypotonia resulting from systemic infection, electrolyte disorders, hypermagnesemia, seizures or drugs administered to the infant or mother and the reduced tone and power of preterm infants are not included in the definition of the hypotonic infant.

Clues from the history

- Family history – may be consanguinity, unexplained deaths.
- May be increasing severity with succeeding generations, e.g. muscular dystrophy.
- Clinical features in mother – ptosis in myasthenia gravis, absence of facial expression and weak grip in myotonic dystrophy and family history of cataracts.
- Pregnancy – polyhydramnios and reduced fetal movements.

Causes and clinical features (Table 58.1)

Table 58.1 Causes and clinical features of central and peripheral hypotoma.

	Central hypotonia	**Peripheral hypotonia**
Causes	Cerebral malformation. Encephalopathy: • Hypoxic–ischemic encephalopathy • Meningitis/encephalitis • Hypoglycemia. Chromosomal/syndromes: • Trisomy 21 (Down syndrome) • Prader–Willi syndrome Metabolic: • Hypothyroidism • Inborn errors of metabolism, e.g. hyperammonemia, amino acidopathy.	Anterior horn cell: • Spinal muscular atrophy (Werdnig–Hoffmann syndrome). Neuromuscular junction: • Neonatal myasthenia gravis. Muscles: • Congenital myopathies • Myotonic dystrophy.
Clinical features	Antigravity movements present. Normal or brisk tendon reflexes. Features of brain dysfunction may be present.	Weak or absent antigravity movements from severe muscle weakness. Reduced or normal tendon reflexes. Other features – see Fig. 58.2.

Investigations

May include:
- karyotype/DNA analysis
- imaging of brain – MRI, CT or ultrasound
- blood glucose, calcium, magnesium and lactate
- acid–base status, urine and plasma amino acids, urine organic acids, plasma ammonia, lactate
- CPK (creatine phosphokinase) – raised in muscular dystrophy
- thyroid function tests

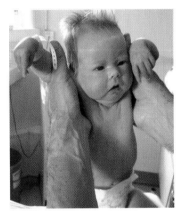

(a)

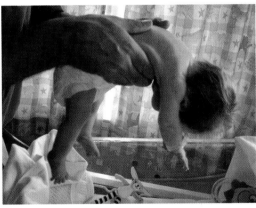

(b)

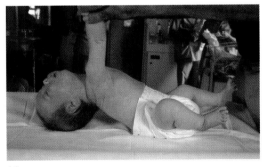

(c)

Fig. 58.1 (a) When held upright, the infant slides through one's hands. (b) When held prone, the infant flops like a rag doll. (c) On traction of the arms, there is marked head lag.

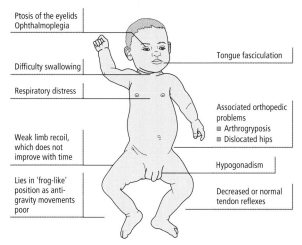

Fig. 58.2 Clinical features that may be present with a peripheral neuromuscular disorder.

Labels in figure:
Ptosis of the eyelids
Ophthalmoplegia
Difficulty swallowing
Respiratory distress
Weak limb recoil, which does not improve with time
Lies in 'frog-like' position as anti-gravity movements poor
Tongue fasciculation
Associated orthopedic problems
  ■ Arthrogryposis
  ■ Dislocated hips
Hypogonadism
Decreased or normal tendon reflexes

- congenital infection screening tests
- EMG (electromyogram)
- muscle biopsy.

Some specific conditions

Central

Hypoxic–ischemic encephalopathy
Hypotonia may be replaced by spasticity when older.

Prader-Willi syndrome
- 70% have partial chromosomal deletion (imprinting from a paternal deletion or uniparental disomy of two maternal chromosomes.
- Characteristic facies (Fig. 58.3).
- Hypotonia.
- Hypogonadism/cryptorchidism.
- Obesity beyond neonatal period.
- Developmental delay.

Peripheral (rare)

Spinal muscular atrophy (Werdnig–Hoffmann syndrome)
- Autosomal recessive – anterior horn cell degeneration.
- Pregnancy – decrease or loss of fetal movements.
- At birth – arthrogryposis (contractures) may be present.
- Characteristic feature – fasciculation of tongue.

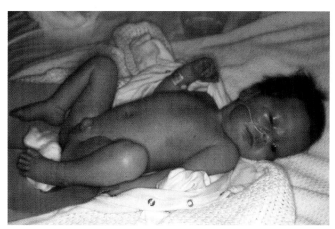

Fig. 58.3 Prader–Willi syndrome. Characteristic facies and hypogonadism. The nasogastric tube is because of poor feeding. (Courtesy of Dr. Mike Coren.)

- Severe, progressive disorder, death from respiratory failure during first year of life.
- DNA test available.

Neonatal myasthenia gravis
- Affects 10–20% of infants of mothers with myasthenia gravis.
- Transient condition, from maternal anti-acetylcholine antibodies.
- Neonate – generalized weakness, facial diplegia, rarely ptosis, weak suck and cry, tendon reflexes normal.
- Use neostigmine, not tensilon, to confirm diagnosis.

Myotonic dystrophy
- Autosomal dominant – inherited from the mother (trinucleotide repeat expansion mutations). Earlier and more severe presentation in successive generations.
- Pregnancy – polyhydramnios and decreased fetal movement.
- Neonate – weakness, edema and petechiae at birth with or without arthrogryposis.
- Facial diplegia, ptosis, tent-shaped mouth, club foot.
- Brain abnormalities present in some forms of muscular dystrophies.
- CPK may be elevated, EMG and biopsy are diagnostic.

Congenital myopathies
- Most are recessively inherited.
- Neonate – weak, hypotonic, areflexic.
- Abnormal swallowing, normal extra-ocular movements.
- Muscle weakness usually slowly progressive.

Congenital abnormalities of the hip and feet

Developmental dysplasia of the hip, DDH (congenital dislocation of the hip, CDH)

Hip is dislocatable, dislocated and/or has shallow acetabulum.

Incidence
- 6 per 1000 livebirths have abnormal clinical examination on screening.
- 1.5 per 1000 livebirths are treated.

Risk factors, clinical examination and initial management
These are described in Chapter 16.

Treatment
- Double diapering (double nappies) – efficacy is questionable.
- Pavlik harness for 1–3 months (Fig. 59.1):
  - maintains flexion and abduction
  - redirects femoral head towards acetabulum.
- Traction, splinting or open reduction and derotation femoral osteotomy may be required.

Outcome
- 80–95% identified on screening do not need surgery.
- 5% of treated cases develop avascular necrosis (ischemic damage) of the femoral head.
- The impact of routine neonatal screening on the need for surgery is uncertain.

Talipes equinovarus

Anatomy
Foot held in rigid equinovarus position (Fig. 59.2a and b). Needs to be distinguished from positional talipes (see Chapter 20).

Incidence
1 in 1000 livebirths.

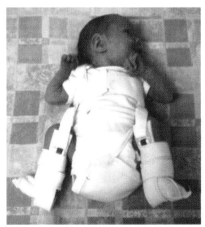

Fig. 59.1 Pavlik harness for treatment of developmental dysplasia of the hip.

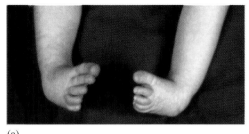

(a)

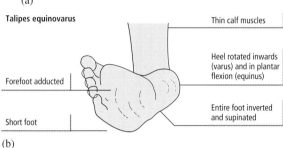

(b)

Fig. 59.2 (a and b) Talipes equinovarus. The foot is inverted and supinated and the forefoot is adducted. The affected foot is shorter and the calf muscles thinner than normal. The position of the foot is fixed and cannot be corrected by passive manipulation.

Risk factors
- Multifactorial inheritance.
- 20–30% risk if affected parent.
- 3% risk for subsequent siblings.
- May be congenital or secondary (teratologic) to:
  - oligohydramnios
  - neuromuscular disorder, e.g. spina bifida
  - malformation syndrome.
- May be associated with developmental dysplasia of the hip.

Management
- Refer to orthopedic surgeon.
- Neonatal treatment – stretching, strapping or serial plaster casts (Fig. 59.3).
- Maximal correction is by 3 months of age.
- Corrective surgery usually required at 6–12 months.

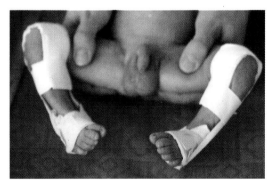

Fig. 59.3 Treatment of talipes equinovarus with serial plaster casts.

Infection

Septic arthritis

- Rare in newborn.
- Usually from extension from underlying bone infection, rather than primary infection of the joint or from hematogenous spread.

Signs

- Decreased joint movement.
- Joint is swollen, warm, red (Fig. 59.4).
- Effusion may be present.

Diagnosis

Joint aspiration for cell count, >50 000 white blood cells/mm^3 (>50 white blood cells × 10^9/L), gram stain, culture, protein, glucose (<30% of serum level).

Imaging

- Ultrasound – fluid in joint space.
- Radionuclide bone scan – hot spot.
  Plain X-ray is of limited value – may show widened joint space.

Treatment

- Single or repeated needle aspiration.
- Surgical drainage of hip joint if no improvement.
- Antibiotics – prolonged course for 3–6 weeks.

Long-term complications

- Erosion of articular surface.
- Joint ankylosis.

Osteomyelitis

- Rare in newborn.
- Most are hematogenous in origin, in metaphysis.
- Usually presents within first 2 weeks of life.

Pathogens

Commonest are *Staphylococcus aureus* and streptococci.

Signs

- No movement (pseudoparalysis) of limb.
- Red, warm, swollen, painful limb.

Diagnosis

- Blood culture positive.
- Bone aspiration for cultures if indicated.

Imaging

- Ultrasound – periosteal elevation and soft tissue swelling.
- Radionuclide bone scan – hot spot (needle aspiration does not produce positive bone scan).
- Plain X-ray – limited use at this stage, as only shows periosteal elevation and soft tissue swelling.
- MRI scan of bone if necessary.

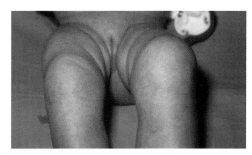

Fig. 59.4 Septic arthritis showing swollen left knee.

Treatment

Antibiotics – prolonged course for 3–6 weeks. Continue for 2–3 weeks after symptoms resolve and ESR (erythrocyte sedimentation rate) or CRP (C-reactive protein) normalizes.

Skeletal dysplasias

There are several hundred, with shortening of the limbs and spine resulting in short stature.

Achondroplasia

- Short bowed limbs, normal trunk, large head.
- Midface hypoplasia, frontal bossing.
- Trident hand (short and broad), protuberant abdomen.

Osteogenesis imperfecta

- Inherited disorder of type 1 collagen formation.
- Rare – 1 in 20 000 live births.

Clinical features

- Increased bone fragility, susceptibility to fracture (Fig. 59.5).
- Blue sclerae, defective tooth formation in some patients.
- Hearing loss.
- Scoliosis, kyphosis.

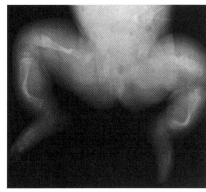

Fig. 59.5 X-ray of osteogenesis imperfecta showing multiple fractures.

Hearing

Congenital hearing loss affects 1–2/1000 live births. If the infant receives neonatal intensive care, risk is increased 10-fold.

Hearing loss is either:
- **conductive** – involves conduction of sound in the middle or outer ear, as usually occurs in childhood from secretory otitis media; or
- **sensorineural** – involves the hair cells of the cochlea in the inner ear, or the cochlear branch of cranial nerve VIII, as in congenital or neonatal hearing loss.

The speech and language of children with severe hearing impairment is delayed or does not develop. The earlier in life hearing can be restored or specialist assistance provided, the better the outcome. Screening infants with risk factors (Table 60.1) identifies only 40–60% of significant bilateral hearing loss. Conventional hearing testing in infants using the distraction test is unreliable and can only be performed at 6 months of age. Universal screening by 3 months of life is therefore recommended (Table 60.2).

Neonatal hearing screening

Can be performed with automated auditory brainstem response (AABR) (Fig. 60.1) or evoked otoacoustic emissions (EOAE) (Fig. 60.2).

Table 60.1 Risk factors for hearing loss.

Family history
Syndromes with hearing loss
Malformations of the ears, including pits and tags
Perinatal
Very low birthweight
Congenital infection – CMV (cytomegalovirus), rubella
Hyperbilirubinemia
Ototoxic medications, e.g. furosemide
Mechanical ventilation – hyperventilation
Hypoxic–ischemic encephalopathy
Bacterial meningitis

Table 60.2 Rationale for universal hearing screening.

Is hearing impairment common?
Relatively – more common than hypothyroidism, phenylketonuria or hemoglobinopathy
Is the condition serious?
Yes. Results in marked speech and language delay
Is treatment available?
Yes. Sound amplification, finger-spelling, lip-reading, using gestures and sign language to maximize early development of language skills
Are reliable screening tests available?
Yes. Somewhat complex, but have acceptable sensitivity and specificity
Are other methods of detection available?
Other methods, e.g. parental concern, are unreliable
Does it improve outcome?
Yes. The earlier amplification and specialist intervention for infant and family the better the outcome
Can it be done at reasonable cost?
Yes, but requires skilled audiology backup for retesting

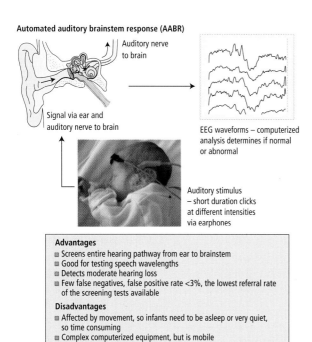

Advantages
- Screens entire hearing pathway from ear to brainstem
- Good for testing speech wavelengths
- Detects moderate hearing loss
- Few false negatives, false positive rate <3%, the lowest referral rate of the screening tests available

Disadvantages
- Affected by movement, so infants need to be asleep or very quiet, so time consuming
- Complex computerized equipment, but is mobile
- Requires electrodes applied to infant's head, which parents may dislike

Fig. 60.1 Automated auditory brainstem response (AABR).

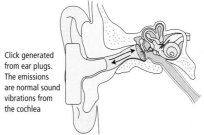

Advantages
- Simple and quick to perform, though is affected by ambient noise

Disadvantages
- Misses auditory neuropathy
- False positive rate of up to 30% in first 24 hours after birth as vernix or amniotic fluid are still in ear canal
  Referral rate of 6–8%, with risk of loss to follow-up
  Can reduce referral rate to 1% by doing AABR if fail EOAE testing but adds complexity to screening program

Fig. 60.2 Evoked otoacoustic emissions (EOAE).

Vision

The normal term infant will fix and follow a moving face or brightly colored object (e.g. a red ball) horizontally. They prefer to look at patterned objects rather than plain ones.

Visual acuity is initially poor – only about 6/200. It improves over the first few months, to 6/60 at 3 months, but adult visual acuity is not reached until about 3 years. At birth, many have mild hypermetropia (far-sightedness), which persists through early childhood; clarity of vision is achieved by accommodation. This contrasts with preterm infants, who are often myopic (nearsighted).

The eyes of newborn infants are often not aligned, and an intermittent squint (strabismus) is common during the first weeks of life. A constant squint persisting beyond 6 weeks of life should be referred to an ophthalmologist.

Lesions needing urgent ophthalmologic referral

During early childhood, failure of focussed visual images to reach the retina, e.g. from a cataract or glaucoma, results in permanent loss of vision (amblyopia). Optimal vision is achieved if surgery and optical correction are performed soon after birth. Affected infants must therefore be referred urgently to an ophthalmologist for surgery.

Cataracts
Cataracts may be detected by parents or on checking the red reflex with an ophthalmoscope during the routine examination of the newborn, but may otherwise present with blindness at several months of age. Many are genetic, but congenital infection and other causes must be excluded.

They are infrequent.

Congenital glaucoma
Intraocular pressure is raised. There is watering of the eyes, photophobia and irritability. The eye becomes enlarged and the cornea hazy. Most are bilateral.

Other congenital abnormalities

There are numerous, rare, congenital abnormalities of the eye, including:
• coloboma (Fig. 60.5)
• aniridia (absence of iris)
• albinism (lack of melanin pigment in iris and retina) – may be ocular or generalized, often resulting in macular hypoplasia, nystagmus and poor vision
• white pupil (leukocoria) or white reflex on ophthalmoscopy – causes include retinoblastoma, cataract, retinopathy of prematurity.

Affected infants should be referred to an ophthalmologist.

The causes of severe visual impairment and blindness in children are listed in Table 60.3. Most visually disabled children also have other disabilities.

Other eye conditions

• Retinopathy of prematurity – see Chapter 34.
• Conjunctivitis – see Chapter 41.
• Choroidoretinitis in congenital infection – see Chapter 10.

Table 60.3 Causes of severe visual impairment and blindness in children (<16 years).

Whole globe and anterior segment	7%
Glaucoma, cornea, lens (cataract)	10%
Congenital infection	2%
Retina	29%
Retinopathy of prematurity	3%
Oculocutaneous albinism	4%
Optic nerve, cerebral/visual pathways	76%

From Rahi *et al*. Severe visual impairment and blindness in children in the UK. *Lancet* 2003; **362**: 1359–65.

Cataract

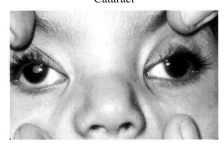

Fig. 60.3 Cataract in right eye of a newborn infant. (Courtesy of Prof. Alistair Fielder.)

Glaucoma

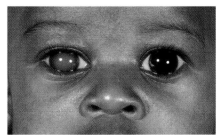

Fig. 60.4 Congenital glaucoma of right eye. (Courtesy of Prof. Alistair Fielder.)

Coloboma

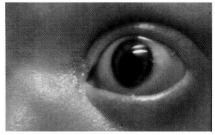

Fig. 60.5 Coloboma. Most often is a keyhole-shaped defect of the iris inferiorly. May also affect the choroid and other structures. Vision may be normal in mild cases, but poor if optic nerve involved.

61 Pain

Pain is a subjective cortical experience. Although it is not possible for a neonate to describe a painful experience to us, there is good evidence from physiologic and behavioral responses that they respond to pain and it causes distress (Table 61.1). Pain is one of the main parental concerns for infants in intensive care or undergoing procedures. They often also worry about long-term consequences. There is evidence that children who undergo repeated painful experiences as neonates show increased sensitivity to pain in childhood, e.g. to an immunization, and are more fearful of pain than their peers.

Development of pain pathways in the fetus and preterm infant

Although it was thought for many years that preterm and newborn infants were unable to feel pain as their nerves were unmyelinated, it has now been shown that at:
- 20 weeks' gestation – sensory receptors and cortical neurons have developed
- 24 weeks – cortical synapses present
- 30 weeks – myelination of pain pathways and development of spinal cord synapses with sensory fibers.

Implications

- Even preterm infants have anatomical, neurophysiological and hormonal components to perceive pain.
- Central descending inhibitory control is less well developed – so response to painful stimuli is actually greater than in older children and adults.

Factors that modify pain responses

Infants requiring intensive care are subjected to an average of two to 10 painful procedures per day. They are also repeatedly disturbed, e.g. for examination, nursing care, etc.

The pain they experience will be affected by:
- procedure being performed (Fig. 61.1), the skill of the operator and their concern about minimizing pain and discomfort
- gestational age and postnatal age
- behavioral state
- number of previous painful experiences
- time since last painful experience
- severity of their illness.

Assessment of pain

Pain can be assessed clinically according to:
- Physiologic responses:
  - heart rate, respiratory rate, oxygen requirement, blood pressure, palmar sweating.
- Behavioral responses:

Table 61.1 Some milestones in neonatal pain.

1987	Thoracotomy for surgical ligation of patent ductus arteriosus – greater physiologic and hormonal responses if performed without analgesia
1990s	Increasing awareness and concern about neonatal pain
2000	American Academy of Pediatrics Policy Statement on Prevention and Management of Pain and Stress in the Neonate
2001	International Consensus Statement for the Prevention and Management of Pain in the Newborn

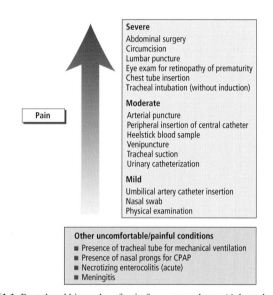

Fig. 61.1 Postulated hierarchy of pain from procedures. (Adapted from Porter F *et al*. Procedural pain in newborn infants: the influence of intensity and development. *Pediatrics* 1999; **104**: 1–10.)

  - facial expression, body movements, crying.
- Metabolic responses:
  - stress hormones, e.g. cortisol
  - blood glucose, lactate.

These may be used as proxy measures of pain. Obtaining reliable results is problematic and their interpretation is difficult.

Pain assessment scales

A variety of neonatal pain assessment scales have been developed (Table 61.2), mainly for clinical research or postoperative pain assessment (CRIES score). The simpler scales can also be used for regular, systematic pain assessment for infants undergoing intensive care, or as guidance for staff on pain assessment.

Minimizing pain

There are both non-pharmacologic and pharmacologic approaches to the management of pain.

Table 61.2 Some pain assessment scales in newborn infants.

Newborn Pain Assessment Scale (NPAS)	Premature Infant Pain Profile (PIPP)	Neonatal Facial Coding Scale (NFCS)	CRIES score
Behavioral cues: • Sleep in preceding hour • Facial expression of pain • Motor activity • Tone • Consolability • Cry Physiologic cues: • Heart rate • Systolic blood pressure • Respiratory frequency and pattern • Oxygen saturation	Gestational age Behavioral state Brow bulge Eye squeeze Nasolabial furrow Heart rate Oxygen saturation	Brow bulge Eye squeeze Nasolabial furrow Open lips Stretch mouth Lip purse Taut tongue Chin quiver Tongue protrusion	**C**rying **R**equires increased oxygen **I**ncreased vital signs **E**xpression **S**leeplessness

Always consider:

- is any procedure really necessary?
- timing the procedure for when the infant is awake, if possible
- grouping procedures together, **but** limit the number of procedures occurring within a short time of each other (as with physical training, we all need recovery time!)
- using equipment or methods designed to minimize discomfort (e.g. appropriate heel lancets, non-invasive monitoring, venous or arterial catheters to avoid repeated skin punctures, avoiding intramuscular injections unless essential, etc.).

Non-pharmacologic

These include:

- environmental modification:
  - talking to baby, stroking, rocking, skin-to-skin contact
- non-nutritive sucking on a pacifier (dummy)
- sucrose pacifiers – high-concentration sucrose shown to reduce pain response
- containment or positioning (Fig. 61.2).

Pharmacologic approaches

Infants on mechanical ventilation

Opioids are the main analgesic agents. In neonates, the most widely used are:

- morphine – also improves synchrony between the infant's breathing and the ventilator – side effects include drop in blood pressure, respiratory depression and abstinence (withdrawal) syndrome if too rapid dose reduction after prolonged use
- fentanyl – side effects include respiratory depression, tolerance, glottic and chest wall rigidity.

Procedures

Optimal analgesia aims to prevent rather than treat pain. In the past, fear of side effects limited the use of opioids and anesthetic agents, but it should now be possible to provide adequate pain relief. Options include:

- opioids – boluses may be required if on continuous opioid infusion

- general anesthesia – all major or surgical procedures
- regional anesthesia – e.g. peripheral nerve blocks, spinal or epidural, local infiltration – increasingly used in neonates for some surgical procedures and postoperative analgesia
- non-opioids – e.g. acetaminophen (paracetamol); sometimes used for a minor procedure or postoperatively.

Question

How can the pain of heelsticks be minimized?

Pain is mainly from squeezing the foot, so keep to minimum. Autostylets less painful than lancets.

Venipuncture less painful and adequate samples obtained twice as often, but not suitable for repeated sampling.

Topical analgesia – not effective for heelsticks and not licensed in US in newborns. Theoretical concern about methemoglobinemia, but not a problem in practice.

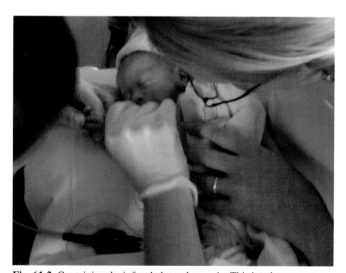

Fig. 61.2 Containing the infant helps reduce pain. This involves secure, supported, non-restrictive positioning, not tight swaddling to prevent moving or extending. Here, during the insertion of a nasogastric tube, the mother is containing her baby and the infant is grasping the nurse's finger.

Pharmacology

The pharmacology of drugs in neonates differs significantly from that in children and adults. In newborn infants there is a huge range in their size, from the extremely preterm, who may weigh only 500 grams, to term infants of 5000 grams, so drug doses vary widely and are prescribed on a mg/kg basis. The wide range in maturity of neonates at birth affects the pharmacokinetics, i.e. the fate of the drug, including absorption, distribution, metabolism and elimination (Fig. 62.1).

The law

There are strict licensing laws governing the use of drugs. However, many drugs used in neonatal care are not licensed (unlicensed drugs) or are used outside the terms of their license (off-label drugs). This is often because it is not commercially viable for pharmaceutical companies to obtain product licenses for neonates. This does not mean that they should not be used, but it imposes additional responsibility on prescribers in neonatal practice to ensure that the currently available evidence supports the use of a particular drug in a specific neonatal situation.

Quality assurance

Quality assurance (clinical governance) is a framework for **accounting** for the quality of clinical services and for their improvement (Fig. 62.3).

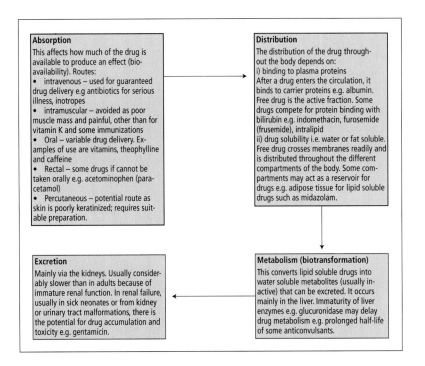

Fig. 62.1 Absorption, distribution, metabolism and excretion of drugs in newborn infants.

Question

What do trough and peak levels indicate?

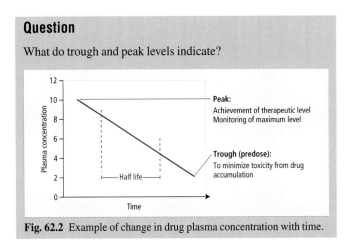

Fig. 62.2 Example of change in drug plasma concentration with time.

Key point

Some prescribing lessons from the past
- Interactions:
  – Sulfonamides displaced bilirubin from albumin and increased risk of kernicterus.
- Side effects:
  – Chloramphenicol was responsible for the 'gray baby' syndrome of circulatory collapse.
  – Topical antiseptics containing iodine can result in hypothyroidism from absorption, so use sparingly and wipe away.

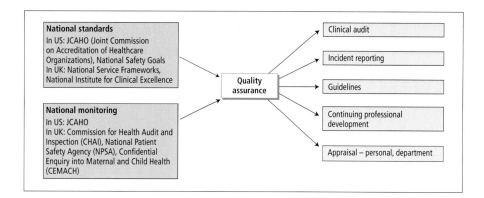

Fig. 62.3 Framework for quality assurance.

Clinical audit

Aims to improve patient care and outcomes through systematic review against explicit criteria followed by change. The audit cycle is shown in Fig. 62.4.

Clinical incident reporting (Table 62.1)

Table 62.1 Questions and answers about clinical incidents.

What are they?	Unexpected events that cause or could cause harm to the patient. Include near-misses
Who should report them?	Everyone
What should be reported?	The facts
Why report?	To identify causes To develop a strategy to prevent recurrence To act as warning for complaints/litigation To provide information for external monitoring
Who is to blame?	A no-blame culture should be developed – disciplinary action will not follow EXCEPT where acts or omissions are malicious, criminal, or constitute gross professional misconduct
What level of investigation is required?	Depends on extent of harm to the patient and assessment of likelihood of recurrence by taking the whole circumstance of the event into account, not just the incident itself If risk of harm or recurrence is high, perform root cause analysis
What is root cause analysis?	Ask why it occurred rather than focussing on the problem
What if major harm has occurred or major damage to the organization?	Because of potential litigation, the hospital risk management group and senior managers should be informed. A more detailed, formal causal analysis (FMEA, failure mode and effect analysis) should be undertaken

The audit cycle (Fig. 62.4 and Table 62.2)

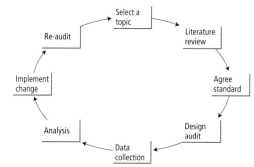

Fig. 62.4 The audit cycle.

Table 62.2 Questions about audit.

Who?	All health professionals
How are topics selected?	Observing current practice Clinical incidents, complaints and claims, etc.
Design?	Agree standards Multidisciplinary Identify data sample Only collect relevant data
Analysis and recommendations	Were standards met? Feedback results Identify improvements Develop an action plan Re-audit to check improvement

A survey in the US showed that medical errors were responsible for 98 000 deaths per year, i.e. more people die in a year in the US from medical errors than from motor vehicle accidents or breast cancer or AIDS.

In a prospective study of pediatric admissions to hospital, potential adverse events were highest in the NICU (neonatal intensive care unit):

- 91% of admissions had a medication error
- 46% of admissions had a potential adverse event
- 74% of errors involved physician ordering.

Neonatal clinical incidents which may relate to fetal or obstetric care will need to be considered in conjunction with maternal–fetal medicine, e.g. hypoxic–ischemic encephalopathy or seizures within 48 hours of birth. Other clinical incidents involving neonatal care are considered within neonatal quality assurance.

The commonest iatrogenic disorders are medication errors and extravasation injuries, but a selection of frequent or important examples follows. Some approaches to their prevention are given, but each clinical incident will need to be considered by the multidisciplinary risk management team.

Prevention of clinical incidents requires a culture of safety throughout the unit (Fig. 63.1).

Extravasation of intravenous infusions (Figs 63.2 and 63.3)

Cause

- Fragile tissues.
- Small catheter, difficult to fix securely.
- Movement by infant.
- Irritant infusion – e.g. calcium, high concentration of dextrose, total parenteral nutrition.

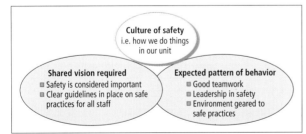

Fig. 63.1 Requirements of a culture of safety in the neonatal unit. (Adapted from J. Horbar, Vermont–Oxford Network.)

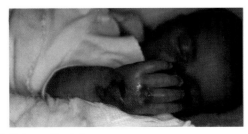

Fig. 63.2 Extravasation injury.

Medication errors

Why?

- Prescription errors occur as there is a wide range of dosage – varies 10-fold if weighs 0.5 kg or 5 kg (unlike adults, where there is usually a standard dose).
- Dilutions often needed – common source of error.
- Use of potentially dangerous drugs – insulin, inotropes, aminophylline, digoxin, narcotics, heparin.

Prevention

- Staff training, with input and checking by pediatric pharmacist.
- Clear formulary.
- Minimize range of drugs used.
- Computer-assisted guidance on dosage and dilutions.
- Avoid abbreviations, e.g. micrograms, not µg.
- Use limited number of standard dilutions, drawn up in pharmacy where possible.
- Clear differentiation between vials, e.g. by color.
- Checking by two trained professionals (but do not rely on this).
- Remove undiluted dangerous drugs, e.g. strong KCl.
- Pay special attention to dangerous drugs.

Prevention

- Expert fixation of catheters.
- Leave potential extravasation area uncovered to be visible.
- Avoid occluding limb with tape.
- Regular checks, pressure-sensitive alarms.
- Give irritant infusions via central lines if possible.

What to do if extensive

- Flush affected area with saline via several skin punctures.
- Consult plastic surgeons if concern about long-term scarring.

Giving wrong breast milk to wrong patient

Cause

- Similar names.
- Poor labeling.

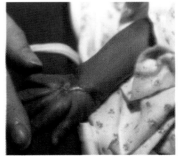

Fig. 63.3 Scarring from extravasation injury.

Prevention

- Clear labeling.
- Double-checking.
- Warning mechanism (name alert tags) for staff if similar names.

Excessive fluid volume infused

Cause

- Incorrect settings on pump.
- Malfunction of pump.

Prevention

- Check and monitor infusion.

Complications of umbilical arterial catheters (UAC)

Incorrect vessel

- Inserted into umbilical vein instead of artery.

Prevention

- Check for presence of arterial pulsation to confirm in artery.
- Check position on abdominal X-ray (Fig. 63.4).

This is important – if in umbilical vein by mistake, excessively high oxygen will be given, which could damage eyes (retinopathy of prematurity, ROP) if preterm.

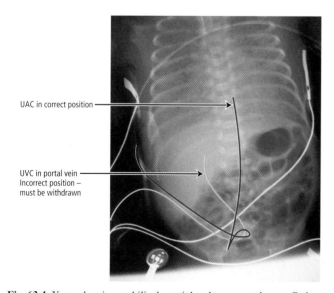

UAC in correct position

UVC in portal vein
Incorrect position –
must be withdrawn

Fig. 63.4 X-ray showing umbilical arterial and venous catheters. Catheter in umbilical artery (red line) – initial course caudally towards groin, then cranially up middle of spine. Catheter in umbilical vein (blue line) – cranial course to right of spine. This catheter is in the portal vein, a potentially dangerous position, and must be withdrawn. In addition, overlapping catheters, as shown here, can easily lead to misinterpretation.

Thrombosis/emboli/vasoconstriction

Consequences

- Occlusion of the artery causes mottling of skin and cyanosis in one or both legs. May result in gangrene/amputation of limb.
- Emboli may affect distant organs.

Prevention

- Regular observation. If skin becomes discolored, reposition or remove catheter.
- Position catheter either high at T6–10 or low at L4–5 to avoid catheter tip near renal vessels to reduce risk of renal artery thrombosis (hematuria, renal failure, hypertension).
- Flush catheter gently, heparinize line.
- Ensure infant's intravascular volume is inadequate.

Blood loss from arterial catheters

Cause

- Disconnection of catheter.

Prevention

- Connections screwed together.
- Pressure-sensitive alarm.

Thrombosis from umbilical venous catheters

Cause

- Catheter in portal vein causing portal vein thrombosis.

Prevention

- Check on X-ray that catheter is in the inferior vena cava and not the portal vein.

Ischemic damage from peripheral artery catheters

Cause

- Small size of vessel.

Prevention

- Choose suitable artery:
  - use radial artery but only if ulnar artery shown to be patent (Fig. 63.5) (See Chapter 73 for Allen test.)
  - avoid superficial temporal artery as can cause ischemia of parietal lobe
  - avoid brachial artery as end artery and occlusion may result in loss of distal limb, and median nerve may be damaged.
- Only use for sampling, not injecting.
- Remove if blanching, other than transient.

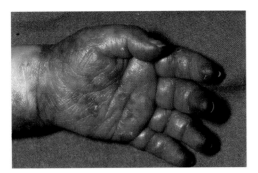

Fig. 63.5 Ischemic damage from radial artery catheter.

Extravasation of total parenteral nutrition (TPN) from central venous lines

Cause

- Catheters may migrate and TPN may be infused into:
  - the tissues, causing swelling and inflammation
  - the lungs, causing pleural effusion
  - the pericardium, causing pericardial effusion and tamponade.

Prevention

- Check catheter tip is in the inferior or superior vena cava, not the right atrium.

Burns and scalds

Cause

- Overheating of humidifier in CPAP/ventilator circuit.
- Disconnection of temperature probe or malfunctioning of radiant warmer (Fig. 63.6).
- Failure to regularly move transcutaneous O_2/CO_2 probes.

Prevention

- Temperature alarms.

Scarring of skin

Cause

- Poorly keratinized skin prone to long-term scarring, especially if Black ethnicity (keloid formation).

Prevention

- Minimize skin damage:
  - care with adhesive tape, probes and pressure from attachments for tracheal tubes, nasal CPAP, etc.

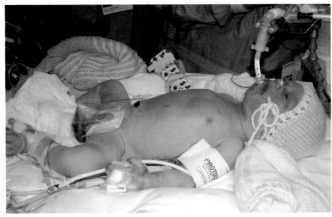

Fig. 63.6 Scalding of skin from excessive heat from radiant warmer on dislodging of skin temperature probe. It resolved within a few hours.

  - if transcutaneous O_2/CO_2 electrodes used, rotate to different skin sites regularly
  - procedures, e.g. chest tube for pneumothorax, incise skin along line of skinfold (Fig. 63.7).

Nasal damage from tracheal tube

Cause

- Dilatation of nostril or damage to the nasal septum by tube.

Prevention

- Avoid excessively large tracheal tubes.
- Avoid leaving in-situ for long periods.
- Fix tube securely to prevent leverage.

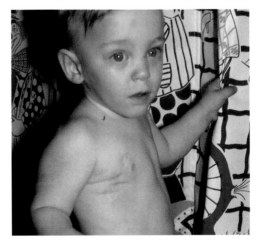

Fig. 63.7 Scarring from chest tubes.

Nasal damage from nasal CPAP

Cause

- Pressure on nostrils or nasal septum.

Prevention

- Correct positioning and distributing pressure over head.

Tracheal stenosis

Cause

- Damage to subglottic area from tracheal tube (Fig. 63.8).

Prevention

- Avoid excessively large tubes.
- Minimize time left in place.
- Secure to prevent tube movement and irritation.

Infection

Cause

- Nosocomial infection – inadequate hand-washing.
- Catheter related – at insertion or subsequently, e.g. breaking of long line.
- Procedures – infection where skin denuded from monitor probes or tape.

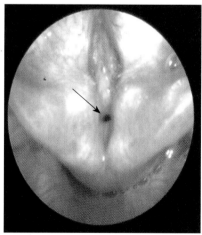

Fig. 63.8 Tracheal stenosis following prolonged mechanical ventilation. The narrowed trachea is shown with an arrow.

Prevention

- **Meticulous hand-washing**.
- Sterile insertion.
- Minimize interference of lines.
- Remove lines as soon as possible.

Aspiration pneumonia from misplaced gavage (nasogastric) feeding tubes

Cause

- Tube inserted into trachea instead of stomach.

Prevention

- Check correct position with pH indicator paper.

Question

Are there any safety initiatives specifically for neonatal care?

Many local and national intiatives, but the most comprehensive dedicated to neonatal care is the Vermont–Oxford Neonatal Intensive Care Quality Network.

It aims to improve the quality and safety of medical care for newborn infants and their families by:
- providing an information resource which also uses material from other disciplines in health-care and other professions, e.g. aviation industry
- providing expert faculty
- promoting four key habits to improve outcome (Fig. 63.9)
- organizing collaborative safety improvement projects, e.g. reducing nosocomial infection, by visits between units or via the internet
- voluntary, anonymous collection of errors on web.

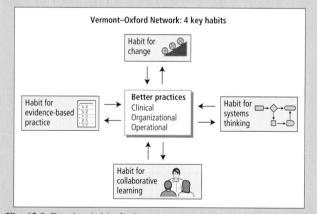

Fig. 63.9 Four key habits for better outcomes promoted by the Vermont Oxford Network. (Reproduced with permission of J. Horbar, Vermont–Oxford Network.)

What is evidence-based medicine (EBM)?

It is the conscientious, explicit and judicious use of current best evidence in making decisions about the care of individual patients.

Steps in the practice of evidence-based medicine

See Fig. 64.1.

Examples of evidence-based medicine in neonatology

The following are some examples from neonatal medicine of therapy proven to be beneficial or harmful. However, for most decisions in clinical practice, guidance from evidence-based medicine is not available, is inconclusive or may be conflicting. Clinicians have to base their decisions on the best available information, clinical experience and the evaluation of potential benefits and risks for the individual patient.

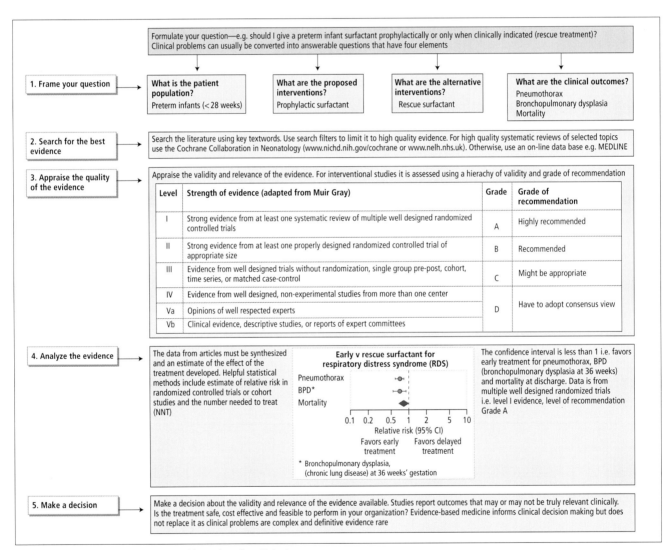

Fig. 64.1 Steps in the practice of EBM (evidence-based medicine).
(Data on surfactant from Yost CC, Soll RF. Early versus delayed selective surfactant treatment for neonatal respiratory distress syndrome (Cochrane Review). In: *The Cochrane Library,* Issue 1, 2004. Chichester, UK: John Wiley & Sons, Ltd.)

Question

What is the effect of antenatal corticosteroids on early neonatal morbidity and mortality in preterm infants?

The meta-analysis (Fig. 64.2) shows that corticosteroids given before preterm birth reduce the incidence of respiratory distress syndrome, intraventricular hemorrhage and neonatal mortality.

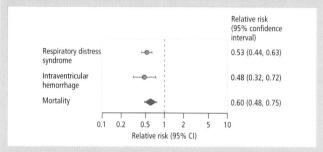

Fig. 64.2 Prophylactic corticosteroids for preterm birth. Data from Crowley P. Prophylactic corticosteroids for preterm birth (Cochrane Review). In: *The Cochrane Library*, Issue 1, 2004. Chichester, UK: John Wiley & Sons.

Beneficial therapies

Examples are:
- Maternal prophylactic corticosteroids for preterm birth.
- Maternal anti-D (Rho) immunoglobulin – to rhesus negative mothers to prevent rhesus disease of the newborn.
- Surfactant therapy in preterm infants.
- Natural versus synthetic surfactant – natural produces greater reduction in ventilator support, fewer pneumothoraces and fewer deaths, but a possible increase in intraventricular hemorrhage (but not for severe hemorrhages).

Harmful therapies

Examples are:
- Uncontrolled oxygen therapy and blindness in preterm infants. This demonstrates the dangers of the introduction of a new therapy, oxygen, followed by changes in its use, without evidence from randomized controlled trials for either change in clinical practice (Fig. 64.4).
- Antibiotic side effects:
    - chloramphenicol (unmonitored) – gray baby syndrome (circulatory collapse)
    - sulfonamides – displacement of bilirubin, resulting in kernicterus
    - tetracycline – yellow staining of teeth and bones.
- Aquaphor, to cover the skin of preterm infants to reduce evaporative heat and water loss – increased risk of sepsis.
- Early prophylactic corticosteroids in preterm infants to reduce severity of respiratory distress syndrome and BPD (bronchopulmonary dysplasia) – gastrointestinal perforation, growth failure, hypertension and possible neurodevelopmental deficit.

Question

What is the effect of the prophylactic surfactant versus no surfactant on early neonatal morbidity and mortality in preterm infants?

The meta-analysis (Fig. 64.3) shows that prophylactic surfactant reduces the incidence of pneumothorax and neonatal mortality; other major complications are unaltered.

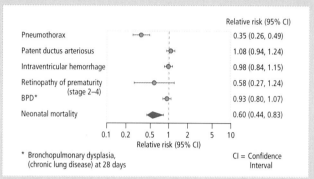

Fig. 64.3 Prophylactic natural surfactant in preterm infants (intubated, <30 weeks). Data from Soll RF. Prophylactic natural surfactant extract for preventing morbidity and mortality in preterm infants (Cochrane Review). In: *The Cochrane Library*, Issue 1, 2004. Chichester, UK: John Wiley & Sons.

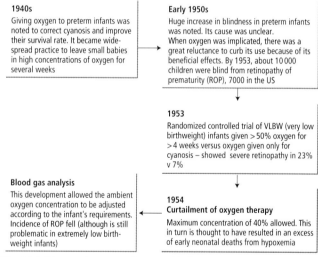

Fig. 64.4 Changes in oxygen therapy with time.

Sick newborn infants have the same rights to life and access to care as any other person. Their care is totally dependent on a successful partnership between parents and the clinical team (Fig. 65.1).

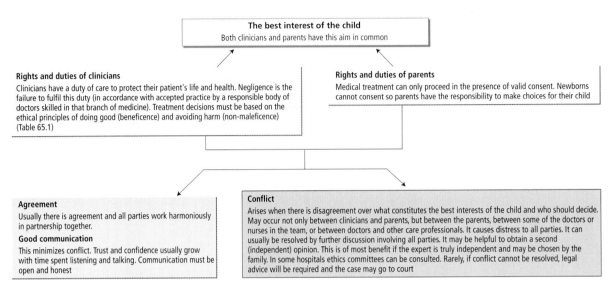

Fig. 65.1 Ethical framework of clinical practice.

Table 65.1 Definitions of the principles of medical ethics.

Beneficence	Do good
Non-maleficence	Do no harm
Justice	Legal justice, respect for rights, fair distribution of resources
Respect for autonomy	Respect for the individuals' right to make informed and thought-out decisions for themselves
Trust	Parents need to develop trust in their physician, who has a responsibility to ensure that this trust is not misplaced

Question

What is the role of clinical ethics committees?

These are increasingly being developed as a resource for doctors and other health care professionals and parents facing difficult ethical problems. Usually include an ethicist, clinicians, lay members, clergy and others, e.g. lawyers, and may include parents. Cases are usually considered in retrospect to inform future ethical decision-making. In the US and some centers in the UK, the committee can also be rapidly constituted to discuss an individual problem proactively. Ethics committees do not have legal responsibility; this rests with physicians. While parents usually have the authority to make decisions on behalf of their children, physicians cannot be compelled to give treatment they do not believe is in the child's best interests. All medical decisions must be transparent, justifiable and clearly documented.

The withholding or withdrawal of life-saving medical treatment

There are a number of situations in neonatal practice where withholding or withdrawal of life-saving medical treatment is considered appropriate (Table 65.2). Their management is influenced by the parents' religious beliefs and cultural background, the laws of the country and national guidelines (e.g. American Academy of Pediatrics, Royal College of Paediatrics and Child Health). These decisions are stressful not only for the parents but also for the health-care team, amongst whom consensus and an agreed management plan should be reached. Consent must be obtained from the parents, but the extent to which they may wish to be involved in the decision-making depends on the individual family. Repeated discussion without coercion may be necessary.

If life-saving support is going to be withheld or withdrawn, all aspects of palliative care including symptom management and psychosocial support should be in place. Many parents will accept the appropriateness of withdrawal of mechanical ventilation and appreciate the opportunity to spend time with their baby away from the technology of intensive care, but with staff to support them. The babies comfort should be a priority and appropriate analgesia and anxiolytics given. Analgesia using opioids should be maintained. Parents need to know that the infant may continue to breathe for some time after disconnection from the ventilator.

If clinical situations do not fit the categories described in Table 65.2 or where there is dissent or uncertainty about the degree of future impairment, the child's life should be safeguarded and full care provided by *all* in the health care team.

Table 65.2 Examples of situations in neonatal practice where withholding or withdrawal of intensive care may be appropriate.

The no hope situation
The child has such severe disease that life-sustaining treatment simply delays death without significant alleviation of suffering, e.g. a child with trisomy 13 or 18 needing mechanical ventilation for congenital abnormalities.

The no purpose situation
The patient may be able to survive with treatment, but it is expected that the degree of physical or mental impairment will be devastating. The child in this situation will never be capable of taking part in decisions regarding treatment or its withdrawal. An example is a newborn with profound neurologic damage following severe hypoxic–ischemic brain damage, in whom microcephaly, profound developmental delay, blindness and quadriplegia are believed to be inevitable.

The unbearable situation
There is progressive and irreversible illness where further treatment is more than can be borne by the infant and family caregivers. An infant with progressive and severe deteriorating respiratory failure from bronchopulmonary dysplasia (chronic lung disease) might be considered in this category.

Questions

What is the difference between withholding and withdrawing intensive care?

There is no ethical or legal distinction between them, though emotionally it may be easier not to start treatment than to withdraw it. If there is uncertainty, provide intensive care and subsequently withdraw it after full assessment.

Is euthanasia allowed?

Giving a medicine with the primary intent to hasten death is unlawful in both North America and Europe (though in the Netherlands it is accepted on a carefully regulated basis). Giving a medicine to relieve pain, which as a side effect may hasten death (the principle of double effect), is ethically appropriate if its primary purpose is to alleviate distress or suffering.

Research

Health professionals wish to provide the best possible care for newborn infants. This should be evidenced-based, but this is only possible when evidence is available from properly conducted research. It is therefore unethical for properly conducted research on newborn infants **not** to be performed. Failure to do research leads to stagnant and second-rate medical care.

Research may be interventional, e.g. evaluation of a new therapy, or non-interventional, e.g. descriptive or observational (Table 66.1).

There are a number of obstacles to overcome in order to perform research in newborn infants. These are practical and ethical.

Practical difficulties in conducting research in infants

These include:
- The number of newborn infants who are preterm or have a specific problem or condition is small and usually requires trials to be multicentered, which adds enormously to the complexity and cost of each study. However, a number of networks have been established to facilitate this, such as the Vermont–Oxford and NICHD (National Institute of Child Health and Human Development) Neonatal Networks, and many multicentered trials have been performed throughout the world (see Cochrane neonatal reviews).
- Funding is difficult to obtain as the number of newborn infants with a specific problem is small, making pharmaceutical companies less likely to develop new products or conduct trials.
- In order to proceed with a trial, the information required about a potential new drug or therapy is becoming ever more stringent. This also applies to pilot studies, making it increasingly difficult to obtain the data required to conduct a larger study.

Ethical difficulties in conducting research in infants

All research must be peer-reviewed and sanctioned by an independent ethics advisory committee – Institutional Review Board in North

Table 66.1 Differences between interventional and non-interventional research.

Interventional (therapeutic) research
Research which directly affects the treatment an individual receives. They may receive a new treatment or, in a randomized trial, a new or conventional treatment or placebo. At the start of the project the answer to the question of which is better will not be known (equipoise).
Use of a placebo instead of treatment is unethical if there is an accepted treatment. The new and potentially better therapy should be compared with accepted treatment.

Non-interventional (non-therapeutic) research
Research that will *not benefit directly* the person involved. This is observational research – e.g. the normal levels of vitamin A in a particular group of infants. The infants themselves will in no way benefit – so the invasiveness of obtaining the information must be minimal (a small extra volume of blood when venipuncture is required for other reasons, or a single venipuncture, well performed with analgesia).

America, local research ethics committee (LREC) and multicentered research ethics committee (MREC), if appropriate, in the UK.

Parents must be able to make informed choices when asked for consent for their infant to take part in research. This can be problematic when decisions need to made rapidly, e.g. when a baby suddenly becomes ill, especially immediately after delivery, when parents are emotionally stressed. The differences between assent and informed consent are outlined in Table 66.2.

Criteria for informed consent for research include:
- **Competence** of the person giving consent.
- **Information** – sufficient for informed choice, including a written information sheet for parents and the use of an interpreter if there are concerns about the parents' understanding of English.
- **Understanding** – parents must have understood the research sufficiently to be able to evaluate choices. In the US and UK, consent can be provided by one parent; in some countries in Europe both parents must agree.
- **Written consent** should be obtained, with one copy for the parents and another filed in the case record.
- **Voluntary** – parents must be aware that they can decline or withdraw from the research without jeopardizing their baby's care.

Consent in clinical practice

Health professionals are under pressure to allow parents greater involvement in decision-making and enable them to give consent to treatment.

Parental consent should be obtained for complex procedures or treatment and for all surgical procedures. Documentation about the communication with the parents explaining the basis, benefits and risks of the procedure or treatment is more important than obtaining a signature on a consent form. Consent for a surgical procedure must be obtained by someone fully conversant with it. However, with infants receiving intensive or special care in a neonatal unit, it would be impractical to obtain detailed consent for the multitude of low-risk procedures performed on their baby. However, parents should be given an overview about what the care of their infant involves and what range of procedures will be performed, both verbally and in an information booklet.

In clinical practice, consent is most problematic about the initial resuscitation and immediate management of extremely premature infants at the limit of viability and when withdrawal of treatment is being considered. The former is considered in Chapter 12 on neonatal resuscitation, the latter in Chapter 65 on ethics.

Question

Is consent required for treatment of acute life-threatening situations?

No, but the clinician must believe that the treatment is in the patient's best interests.

Table 66.2 Informed consent and assent in research.

Informed consent	Agreement in principle (assent)
This comes from the ability to evaluate options in the exercise of choice. It is based on judgment of risk and benefit, which must be made clear by the researcher. It is acknowledged that time (in most normal situations 24 hours) should be allowed between the provision of the information and the decision-making by the parents.	Patients for certain clinical trials must be recruited within minutes or hours of presentation, e.g. research into the best way to ventilate a newborn infant or hypothermia after hypoxic–ischemic encephalopathy. It will be impossible in these situations for parents to assess the trial in a fully informed way. At this emergency stage they should be asked to assent to the trial and their acceptance or otherwise should be recorded in the notes. Formal consent should be obtained over the next hours or days. Assent should only be used where a 24-hour assimilation period cannot be used, and should be sanctioned specifically by the review board/ethics committee when considering the trial protocol.
Fully informed consent is probably never truly possible, but consent should be *sufficiently informed*. Parents should be informed about minor side effects if common and serious ones even if rare. The amount of information exchanged should be appropriate for the situation. An excessive amount of information may confuse.	

In the newborn nursery, most deaths are of extremely preterm infants receiving intensive care, but some are term infants with hypoxic–ischemic encephalopathy, major congenital malformations or metabolic disorders. In the past many of these deaths occurred shortly after birth, but now they often occur after many difficult days or weeks, making the death even more stressful for both parents and staff. When it is expected that the baby is going to die, a management plan is required to ensure optimal symptom control for the infant and psychologic and spiritual support for the parents, siblings and family, and that practical needs before and after death are provided for.

Whenever death is expected, the baby should be in a private area with the family. Occasionally, if desired by the family and community support is available, babies may be allowed to die in the family's home.

Symptom control

The aim is to allow the baby to die free of pain and discomfort and with dignity. Analgesia should not be reduced or discontinued for fear that it might contribute to the infant's death. If mechanical ventilation is withdrawn, extremely preterm infants usually die shortly afterwards, but mature infants may continue to breathe for some time. The parents and family need to be forewarned.

Psychologic and spiritual support for the parents, siblings and family

Frequent and honest discussions should be held about the impending death of the baby between the family and health-care team. This may include grandparents, siblings and other family members.

Grief is the normal response to an infant's death. Parents and staff need to know that it is normal to show their emotions at such a sad time.

Arrange for religious leaders to visit if wanted. Parents may want the baby blessed or baptized.

Practical aspects before and after death

Allow parents and family members to hold the baby before death and afterwards, if desired (but do not force them). Many parents value photos of them and their baby at this time, especially if this is the first occasion they can hold their baby free of tracheal tubes and lines and monitors.

Give unhurried, sympathetic care of the body after death, and provide unrestricted access for parents and visitors.

After the infant has died, provide the family with pictures and personal items – name tags, locks of hair, footprints, etc., of the baby.

Provide information about registering the baby's death and funeral arrangements.

Inform family practitioner, health visitor, obstetrician and other health professionals involved.

Some units have remembrance books and hold memorial services.

Provide information about professional resources and self-help groups for bereavement support and counseling.

After the infant's death

Grief may manifest with shock and disbelief, often followed by anger and guilt. There may be associated physical symptoms of anxiety, depression, tearfulness, loss of appetite, fatigue, insomnia and inability to concentrate. It may last many years but is usually most intense in the first few months. Parents may need advice about supporting siblings, grandparents and other family members in their grief. The two parents may also have different patterns of grief and this may place additional stress on their relationship.

Families often find it helpful to have ongoing communication with the health-care team. A meeting is usually scheduled 4–8 weeks later to provide an opportunity to discuss again the circumstances around the infant's death and to answer any questions about their baby's care, as well as covering any unresolved issues. It may be helpful if the obstetrician is also present. Health-care providers must be good listeners, not lecturers, at these meetings in order to learn how the family is feeling.

If there are concerns about abnormal grieving, referral for professional assessment and assistance can be recommended.

Caring for the staff

The death of a baby can also be deeply upsetting for staff. Many babies who die on neonatal units have needed protracted periods of intensive care, during which time the staff and parents become closely involved in the infant's day-to-day care. They are also likely to have encountered critical periods in the infant's condition which they have overcome together. The infant's death may be perceived as a failure, staff often feeling that the baby might have survived if something had been done differently.

Open discussion between all members of staff both before and after the baby's death is crucial, so that all are fully informed and aware of the situation and are able to express their feelings and concerns. Close dialogue is especially important when withdrawal of care is being considered. Many units also provide personal psychologic support for staff if desired.

Autopsy

Why is it performed?

In some situations, autopsy is a legal requirement, e.g. after a sudden unexpected death, surgery, or if any unnatural causes are implicated. Usually, it is performed to provide feedback for:
• parents, to help them understand why their baby died, and for genetic counseling and planning future pregnancies
• clinicians – to audit their management with a view to future improvement; it may confirm correct or missed diagnoses or complications.

Autopsy also contributes to medical education and research.

It should be performed by a pediatric pathologist.

Comparing clinical and autopsy findings reveal major differences are present in 10–12% and lesser differences in 17–32%.

What does it involve?

Autopsy examination involves:
• Photographs and imaging
  – Photographs form permanent documentation for the patient record. Particularly helpful for dysmorphology.
  – X-rays (and MRI if indicated) for bone and other pathology not evident on clinical examination.
• External and internal examination
  – Involves full-length incision from neck to pubis and over back of head; when sutured afterwards not visible when clothed. All organs are removed and inspected and weighed.
• Histology
  – Widespread samples taken for tissue blocks and slides. Traditionally archived for future reference and studies.

• Organ retention
  – Retained for fixing – mainly brain and heart. Can be reviewed with relevant clinicians. Some retained for teaching and research.

Consent

Detailed consent must be obtained unless the autopsy is legally required. All procedures involved must be described, and agreement reached about whether tissues, slides and organs are retained, disposed of in a lawful and respectful way, or when and how the tissues can be returned for burial. Even if autopsy is legally required, parents should be informed about the procedure.

Why has the autopsy rate fallen?

In the UK autopsy rates fell from over 70% in the 1980s to 40% in 1999, and since then has declined further. There has been a similar decline in the US. In the UK this has largely been due to the public outcry following the revelation that tissue and organ retention without consent was a routine part of the autopsy examination. Particularly contentious was the retention of organs, large numbers of which were stored in some hospitals.

Are there alternatives to autopsy?

MRI-assisted biopsy of target organs has been advocated, but some causes are likely to be missed, e.g. infection and metabolic disorders. Limited autopsy or biopsy confined to specific tissues may be performed, but conventional autopsy remains the gold standard.

68 Discharge from hospital

Taking home a preterm baby who required intensive care and many weeks in a neonatal unit is often daunting for parents (Fig. 68.1).

Their fears are shared by parents of term infants who have become seriously ill or have complex problems.

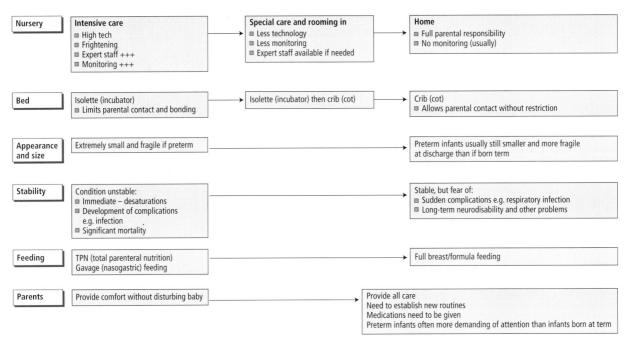

Fig. 68.1 Transition from intensive care to home.

Questions

When can babies go home?

Most go home when their condition is stable and they have established feeding. Parents must be able to care for the baby and provide health-care needs.

Some babies requiring long-term oxygen therapy, e.g. for BPD (bronchopulmonary dysplasia, chronic lung disease), or gavage (tube) feeding can be managed at home (Fig. 68.2).

This depends on the infant's medical condition (likely time course, if otherwise stable, etc.), the parents, home circumstances and community support available.

Should babies with bronchopulmonary dysplasia (chronic lung disease) have a 24-hour saturation recording done before going home?

This is performed in some units a few days after oxygen therapy is stopped to confirm the absence of significant desaturations. Its value has not been established.

All infants who were preterm should be checked to ensure that they are able to maintain their airway and saturations when placed in a car seat.

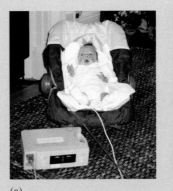
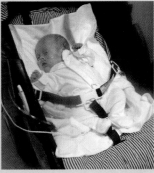

(a)   (b)

Fig. 68.2 (a) Infant receiving oxygen therapy at home, and an oxygen saturation monitor. (b) Same infant receiving oxygen therapy in a stroller.

Discharge planning

Good discharge planning aims to minimize parental anxiety and ensure seamless transfer of care between professionals in the hospital and community. This can be achieved by:
- having a named nurse with this responsibility
- considering discharge arrangements (Fig. 68.3) during regular updates with parents and, if necessary, arranging predischarge meetings with the parents and other professionals involved, e.g.

the family's pediatrician or family practitioner, community nurses, health visitors, therapists, child development team.

Facilities where parents can room in with their baby for several days or longer ('step-down units') before going home are helpful, especially when establishing full breast-feeding.

Some units have specialist nurses who provide care in the family's home and liaise with community-based services. Some of these nurses also work on the unit and know the baby and family before discharge.

Health promotion
i) SIDS (sudden infant death syndrome) prevention:
- Lie on back not prone
- Avoid overheating
- Avoid smoking near baby
ii) Resuscitation training:
- Demonstration, may be complemented by video

Medications
What to give, how often, how to give them and for how long

Immunizations
Which have been given, when are the next ones due?
Is **RSV (respiratory syncytial virus) prophylaxis** (palivizumab, a monoclonal antibody) indicated?
If so, who will give it and when?

Follow-up arrangements
Who, when and where

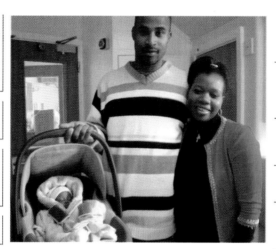

Past and potential medical problems
Check that parents have good understanding
Parents should have a copy of the **discharge summary** in case professional help is needed

Ongoing or new medical problems
Who to contact and how to manage them
Awareness of most likely problems requiring hospitalization, e.g. respiratory infections, inguinal hernias

Feeding
Is breast milk fortifier or a preterm formula feed required?
If so, how can they be obtained and for how long?

Vision and hearing
Have they been checked? Are further checks required?

Parent support group
Would it be helpful, e.g. multiple births, etc? If so, do parents have contact address or is there a helpful internet site?

Fig. 68.3 Parents and their baby leaving the neonatal unit. The items that need to be considered prior to discharge are listed.

Goals

The goals of high-risk follow-up are:
- early identification of disability or developmental or behavior problems
- management of ongoing medical problems related to their neonatal course
- facilitation of early intervention, with referral if necessary
- family support
- monitoring of neonatal outcomes.

Criteria

High-risk infants include:
- preterm (<1500 g or <32 weeks of gestation)
- neurologic abnormality – clinical or imaging
- neonatal seizures
- abnormal neurologic examination at discharge
- hypoxic–ischemic encephalopathy
- mechanical ventilation/nitric oxide therapy/ECMO
- neonatal meningitis
- severe IUGR (intrauterine growth restriction)
- congenital malformations (significant)
- maternal drug abuse
- significant parental psychosocial problems.

Organization and timing

Timing of visits will vary with different programs and with the extent of pediatric neurodevelopmental expertise available to the family locally. It will also depend on whether neurodevelopmental outcome is being monitored at standard times. A typical program for clinic visits and reason for their timing is shown in Fig. 69.1.

Who should conduct neonatal follow-up?

Many neonatologists provide neonatal follow-up. This has the advantage of continuity of care for the parents. It also gives direct feedback on the sequelae of neonatal care.

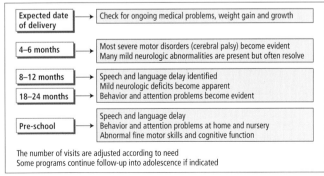

The number of visits are adjusted according to need
Some programs continue follow-up into adolescence if indicated

Fig. 69.1 An example of a high-risk follow-up program.

Multidisciplinary care is required. This includes:
- Developmental specialists – particularly for older children, when developmental assessment and management become more specialized and complex. In some programs all follow-up is performed by developmental specialists.
- Community nursing team – if involved with the family following discharge.
- Dietitian.
- Therapists/child development team.
- Psychologist.
- Social services.
- Family practitioner/pediatrician – provides general pediatric care.

Components

- Growth.
- Neurologic assessment.
- Developmental assessment including behavior.
- Vision and hearing.
- Social/family integration.

Outcome measures

A range of outcomes can be measured (Table 69.1), depending on the purpose of the program or of studies being conducted.

Some specific developmental assessment tools for young children

The most widely used are:
- Bayley scales of infant development 0–3.5 years (Table 69.2)
- Gesell schedules 0–5 years

Table 69.1 Outcome measures

Survival	Functional outcomes:
Medical morbidity	Health or illness
Growth failure	Activity and skills of daily living
Bronchopulmonary dysplasia	Ambulation
(chronic lung disease)	Need for technological aids (gastric
Rehospitalization	tube, oxygen)
Neurodevelopmental outcomes:	Need for special services
Cognitive deficits	Quality of life
Seizure disorder	Impact on family
Cerebral palsy, hyper/hypotonia,	Cost of care
clumsiness	
Hydrocephalus	
Visual impairment	
Hearing impairment	
Behavior disorders	
Special educational needs	

- Griffiths test (in UK) 0–2 years.

For school-aged children:

- Detailed psychometric tests by educational psychologists.

Many premature infants, despite normal neurologic exam and developmental quotient, have special educational needs.

Table 69.2 Bayley scales of infant development.

Subscores	Mental developmental index (MDI)
	Psychomotor developmental index (PDI)
Mean score	100 (standard deviation 15)
Delay	More than 1 standard deviation below the mean (i.e. <85)

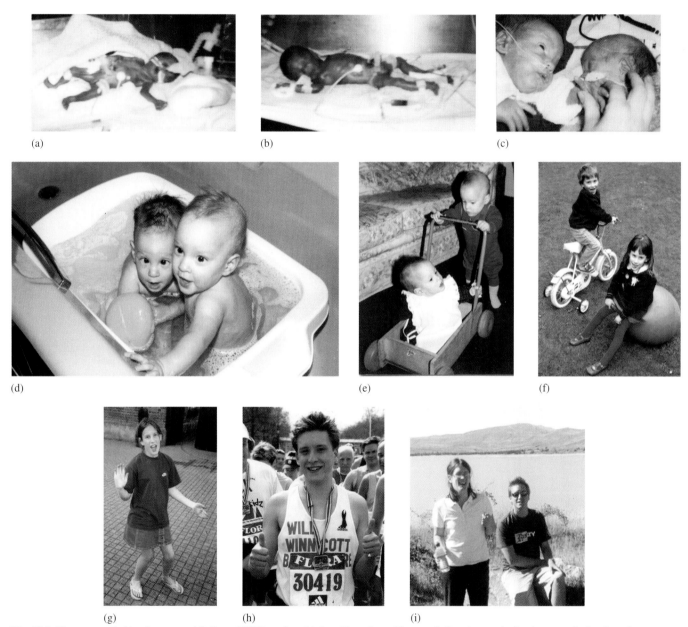

Fig. 69.2 Tiny preterm babies do grow up! Sally and William, from birth at 26 weeks to 19 years. Sally, who required an intraventricular shunt for hydrocephalus, is now learning design; William is at Leeds University studying history. (a) Sally at a few hours in intensive care. (b) William shortly after extubation. (c) Together at last at 4 weeks! (d) At a year. (e) Just walking. (f) At 5 years. (g) Sally at 12 years. (h) At 18 years, William completing the London marathon. (i) At 19 years, on vacation in New Zealand. (With thanks to Sally and William for permitting the use of these photographs.)

Globally, every year there are about:
- 4 million neonatal deaths (Fig. 70.1)
- 4 million stillbirths.

The main causes of neonatal death are shown in Fig. 70.2. About 40% die in the first 24 hours.

Neonatal care in developing countries

Although there has been a marked decline in mortality rates for infants and children less than 5 years old over the last 20 years, neonatal mortality has remained relatively unchanged. This is particularly regrettable as most newborn infants need only primary care, called by the World Health Organization 'essential newborn care'. This comprises:
- basic care at birth
- clean delivery practices
- temperature maintenance – dry baby at birth, keep warm with skin-to-skin contact, warm environment, cover baby, including head
- infection control – clean cutting and tying of cord to prevent neonatal tetanus, prophylactic eye care, immunizations
- exclusive breast-feeding – starting within 1 hour of birth and avoiding any formula milk
- early detection of problems and appropriate care-seeking. Requires families to be informed and have access to health facilities. This is often impeded by strong cultural pressure on mothers and newborn babies not to go outside their home for the first 4–6 weeks.

Low birthweight infants may need additional support with basic resuscitation, warmth, feeding, infection and other complications. Very few infants require high technology neonatology.

An example of how the need for essential newborn care remains unmet in many developing countries is shown in Table 70.1.

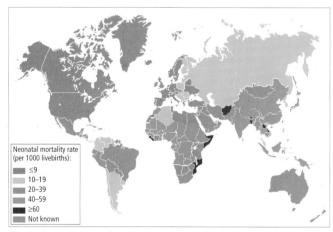

Fig. 70.1 Global overview of neonatal mortality showing 30-fold difference between some countries in sub-Saharan Africa and developed countries.

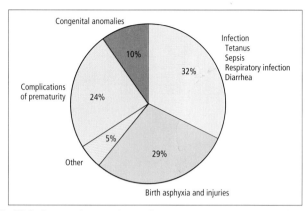

Fig. 70.2 Causes of neonatal mortality. The commonest cause is infection. 19% of all infants are low birthweight; this contributes 40–70% of neonatal deaths.

Table 70.1 Summary of survey of newborn care in rural Nepal, where the neonatal mortality is 50/1000 live births.

90%	Gave birth at home
6%	Skilled attendant at delivery
11%	Alone at delivery
33%	Cord cut with household sickle
64%	Wrapped baby only at 30 minutes of age
92%	Bathed in first hour (high risk of hypothermia)
99%	Breast-fed (Fig. 70.3).

Adapted from Osrin D *et al.*, Cross sectional, community based study of care of newborn infants in Nepal. *BMJ* 2002; **325**: 1063.

Maternal health and obstetric care

Also have a substantial impact on neonatal morbidity and mortality. Priorities in developing countries are:
- before conception
  - birth spacing – considerable health advantages for infant and mother if 3-year birth intervals and mother over 18 years of age
  - nutrition – including calories, protein, iodine, folic acid, iron
  - infection control – malaria, tetanus, sexually transmitted diseases, HIV
- during pregnancy – antenatal care, management of complications
- labor and delivery – skilled attendance, management of complications.

Breast-feeding

Plays a crucial role in prevention of infection and should be strongly encouraged (Figs 70.3 and 70.4).

Breast milk should also be used for low birthweight infants.

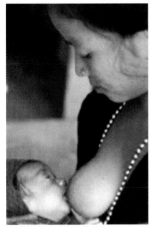 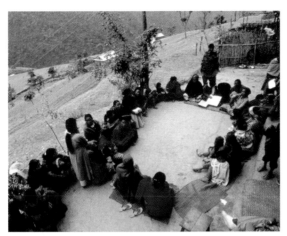 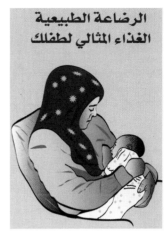

Fig. 70.3 Rural Nepal. (a) Mother breast-feeding. (b) Health education classes for mothers. (Courtesy of Professor Anthony Costello.)

Fig. 70.4 Promotion of breast-feeding in Oman. (Courtesy of Dr Saleh Al-Khusaiby.)

Key point

The promotion and marketing of formula is restricted by the International Code of Marketing of Breast Milk Substitutes (WHO, UNICEF).

HIV infection

Maternal HIV-positive prevalence is as high as 30–40% in many sub-Saharan African countries. This is having a devastating effect on infants and children, who may be infected by vertical transmission and become ill. Not only infected but also non-infected siblings suffer from their parents becoming ill and dying, and having to be cared for by relatives or friends or in institutions.

Many countries are introducing short-course antiretroviral therapy to HIV-positive mothers before delivery.

HIV-positive mothers should breast-feed unless formula feeds can be given safely. Mixed formula and breast-feeding should be avoided, as the risk of transmission appears greater than breast-feeding alone.

Priorities for doctors returning to developing countries after training in developed countries

Most important are:
• measures to prevent infection, e.g. hand hygiene and gloves
• thermal regulation – warm nursery, clothing and hat for infant

• adequate disposable items, e.g. feeding tubes, cannulae
• simple equipment that can be easily operated and maintained, e.g. CPAP
• non-invasive equipment, e.g. pulse oximeters.

However, initial emphasis is often on ventilators and isolettes (incubators). Whilst this may be appropriate in some large centers, for most it is inappropriate because of:
• lack of trained staff
• inability to maintain the equipment
• risk of infection from invasive procedures
• lack of resources.

Questions

Why has neonatal mortality in developing countries failed to decline?

Many reasons, including:
• Neonatal care is often considered 'high-tech'.
• Neonatal care depends on both maternal and child health teaching programs and often falls between them.

How can neonatologists in developed countries help developing countries?

They can help by:
• advocacy – promoting newborn care
• collaborative skills programs – must be adapted for local conditions but still retain scientific rigor and evidence base.

Transport

The infrastructure
- Training – physicians, nurses, respiratory therapists (in US).
- Maintain dedicated equipment.
- A 'transport hotline' – for communication with referring hospitals. Mobile phones for the team on the move.
- Contracts and protocols for transport – ambulance, helicopter (Fig. 71.1), fixed-wing plane (Fig. 71.2).
- Insurance liabilities to cover adverse events.
- Outreach training to less specialized units.

Why transfer?
Higher level of care:
- Prematurity, low birthweight.
- Respiratory distress/failure.
- Intravenous fluids, feeding.
- Sepsis/shock.
- Severe congenital anomalies.
- Hypoxic–ischemic encephalopathy.
- Seizures.
- Hemolytic disease/jaundice.
- Resistant hypoglycemia.
- Metabolic disease.
- Undefined sick infant.
  For subspecialty care:
- Cardiac, surgery, neurosurgery, orthopedic.

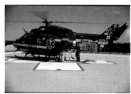

Fig. 71.1 Helicopter transfer in Northern Canada.

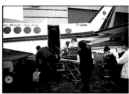

Fig. 71.2 Transport incubator being loaded into fixed-wing plane.

Equipment
- Transport incubator.
- Airways – mask, oral, nasal, tracheal.
- Respiratory support – ventilator, air, oxygen, nitric oxide.
- Full ICU monitoring.
- IV access – infusions, pumps.
- Chest and pericardial tubes.
- Medications.
- Hand-held blood testing – glucose, electrolytes, hemoglobin, blood gases.
- Power source – ambulance, aircraft, hospital wall supply. Battery if nothing else.
  All this is heavy: needs handling skills and equipment to assist.

Initial communication
- Record all clinical details necessary to plan the retrieval.
- Give appropriate advice for ongoing care:
  – Ensure current vital signs, laboratory tests and blood gases are appropriate.
  – Request respiratory support, vascular access, infection treatment, specialist care for cardiac or surgery to be initiated if necessary.
- Request that referring hospital prepares:
  – full documentation of pregnancy, birth and postnatal course; radiographs; laboratory results; vitamin K status.
  – names of baby, parents and contact details.
  – consent for planned procedures.
  – maternal blood for crossmatch.
- Record exact location of patient, city, hospital, ward.
- Estimate arrival time and inform referring hospital.
- Provide ongoing contact number for clinical advice from specialist if needed.

Documentation
- Use standardized clinical assessment and treatment records.
- Necessary for debriefing, audit, legal records.

Key points

Parents need information, support, transport, accommodation, finance, child care and counseling.
  They will remember this experience for the rest of their lives.

Managing the infant

Diagnosis and assessment

- Identify problems and diagnoses needing pretransport therapy.
- Determine the appropriate destination for the identified specialist care needs.

Stabilize before *not during* transport

Baby should have:
- normal temperature
- secure airway and breathing
- optimized blood pressure, circulation, urine output
- optimized blood results – glucose, electrolytes, complete blood

count (CBC), blood gases, etc.
- immediate treatment given, e.g. antibiotics, transfusion, prostaglandin (prostin), anticonvulsants
- status rechecked after transfer to transport incubator.

Access

Tailor to the infant's needs:
- secure airway
- IV access – two lines preferable
- arterial access
- naso/orogastric tubes
- monitoring attached.

Transport

Plan the transfer of the infant over to the transport equipment. Check infant is stable.
- Continuous monitoring, record vital signs regularly as in ICU (Fig. 71.3).
- Keep emergency medications, chest tubes, airways and IV lines accessible.
- Avoid all unnecessary interventions.

Arrival at receiving hospital

Full report to receiving staff.
- Ensure stable transfer to ICU monitoring and therapy.
- Complete documentation.

Aeromedical considerations

- May be faster if ground transport takes more than 2 hours.
- Helicopter maximum distance is about 300 miles, then use fixed-wing plane.
- Local conditions will determine the choice.

Problems:
- Expensive.
- Multiple transfers between vehicles.
- Cramped space/difficult access to baby (Fig. 71.4).
- Noise and vibration.
- Decreased barometric pressure:
  - Fixed-wing planes are pressurized at 8000 ft (2500 m), so, for example, 50% FiO_2 at ground level will require 67% at 8000 ft (2500 m). Prone position may help.
  - There will be expansion of closed air-filled cavities, so:
    - stomach and bowel need a gastric tube
    - pneumothoraces may become more severe
    - blood pressure cuffs may cause occlusion.

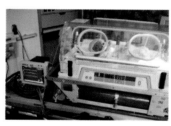

Fig. 71.3 Full monitoring during transport.

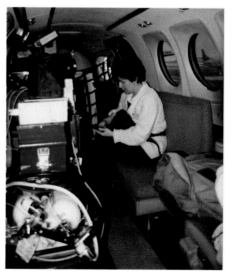

Fig. 71.4 Cramped space in fixed-wing plane.

Endotracheal intubation

Indications

- Neonatal resuscitation (see Chapter 12):
  - failure to respond to clearing of airway, mask ventilation and circulatory support
  - aspiration of meconium.
- Apnea – prolonged/recurrent.
- Increasing work of breathing on CPAP.
- Respiratory failure – defect in oxygenation (hypoxemia) and/or in carbon dioxide elimination (hypercarbia) on CPAP.
- Circulatory failure.
- Administration of surfactant.
- Upper airway obstruction.
- Congenital diaphragmatic hernia.

Procedure

- Place head in neutral position. Insert laryngoscope with left hand to just beyond base of tongue.
- Lift entire blade and identify glottis and epiglottis (Fig. 72.1). Suction if needed.
- Insert tracheal tube (Table 72.1) with right hand into right side of infant's mouth and pass thru the vocal cords (Fig. 72.2) to the level of the cord guide (a black line near the tube tip). A stylet may help in directing the tube through the cords.
- Note depth of insertion from gum or lip.

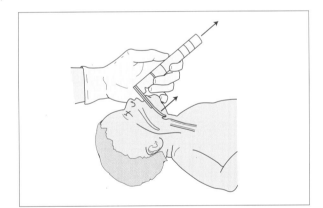

Fig. 72.1 With tip of blade at base of epiglottis, lift the entire blade to visualize the vocal cords. Cricoid pressure may help.

Table 72.1 Endotracheal tube size

Size (mm)	Weight (kg)	Gestation (weeks)	Depth of insertion (cm from upper lip)
2.5	<1	<28	6–7
3.0	1–2	28–34	8
3.5	2–3	35–38	9
3.5–4	>3	>38	10

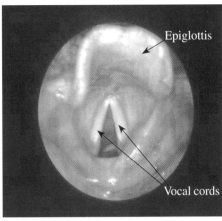

Fig. 72.2 View of vocal cords at intubation.

- Verify placement by positive pressure ventilation, auscultating over upper lungs and stomach. Watch for chest rise with no gastric distension and improvement in heart rate and clinical condition.
- Secure tube, noting any change in tube depth of insertion.
- **Limit attempts to 20–30 seconds.**
- Mask-ventilate and oxygenate infant between attempts.

Nasotracheal intubation

- Advantage – tube stability.
- Disadvantage – risk of nasal damage.

Procedure

- Position infant.
- Insert lubricated nasotracheal tube into nostril to back of throat.
- Insert laryngoscope to visualize vocal cords.
- Using McGill forceps if necessary, advance tracheal tube thru cords.

Elective tracheal intubation

Infants should be given rapid sequence induction before elective intubation, e.g. for surgery:
- muscle relaxant – suxamethonium
- analgesia/anesthesia – morphine or fentanyl
- vagal tone blockade – with atropine, may be indicated.

Mechanical ventilation

Conventional ventilation

Initial ventilator settings

Determined by:
- reason for ventilation, e.g. respiratory distress syndrome, meconium aspiration, PPHN (persistent pulmonary hypertension of

Table 72.2 Typical initial settings on conventional ventilator for respiratory distress syndrome (with range)

FiO$_2$	Minimum for satisfactory oxygen saturation
PIP	18 cm H$_2$O (16–30)
PEEP	4 cm H$_2$O (4–6)
Rate	50 (20–60) breaths/minute
Inspiratory time	0.35 (0.3–0.5) seconds

newborn), pneumonia, normal lungs for apnea, etc.
• size, gestational age and postnatal age – the larger and more mature the infant, the higher the peak pressures.

General principles

Minimize ventilator-induced lung injury (inflammation, air leaks) by:
• using optimal lung expansion:
– avoid lung overexpansion from too high mean airway pressure (volutrauma)
– avoid ventilating underexpanded atelectatic lung (sometimes called atelectotrauma).
• synchronizing ventilator with the infant's breathing – sedation, matching their rates or with patient-triggered ventilation.

Target arterial blood gases

• PaO$_2$: 45–75 mm Hg (6–10 kPa).
• PaCO$_2$: 35–55 mm Hg (4.5–7 kPa).
• pH: 7.25–7.4.

Causes of deterioration of blood gases

SUDDEN DETERIORATION
• Tracheal tube blocked/displaced.
• Ventilator/circuit disconnected or malfunction.
• Air leak – tension pneumothorax or pneumomediastinum.
• Pulmonary hemorrhage.
• Hemorrhage – intraventricular or other sites.

GRADUAL DETERIORATION
• Increased lung secretions.
• Infection.
• Patent ductus arteriosus.
• Anemia.
• Developing bronchopulmonary dysplasia (chronic lung disease).

Abnormal blood gases

Requires:
• check infant – for satisfactory chest wall movement, bilateral air entry, no pneumothorax (transilluminate chest if necessary), airway is clear, and ventilator functioning correctly.
• check breathing is synchronous with ventilator.
• check circulation.
• adjust ventilator settings if necessary.
• recheck blood gases after 20 minutes. Adjusting the ventilator is facilitated by continuous monitoring PaO$_2$ and PaCO$_2$ transcutaneously or by umbilical artery catheter electrode.

Adjusting the ventilator

OXYGEN
Aim is to avoid:
• hypoxemia as it may cause ischemic damage
• hyperoxia in preterm infants as it may cause retinopathy of prematurity.
To improve oxygenation, options are:
• increase inspired oxygen concentration
• increase mean airway pressure – increase PIP, PEEP or inspiratory time (Fig. 72.3).

CARBON DIOXIDE
• Keep PaCO$_2$ in normal range during first 72 hours – to keep cerebral blood flow in normal range during time of maximum risk of intraventricular hemorrhage. Thereafter, allow somewhat higher levels of PaCO$_2$ (permissive hypercapnia) to minimize ventilator-induced lung injury, but keep pH above 7.25.
• Avoid low PaCO$_2$ (<30 mm Hg, 4 kPa) – lowers cerebral blood flow and is associated with ischemic brain injury (periventricular leukomalacia).
To reduce PaCO$_2$:
• increase respiratory rate (but allow sufficient expiratory time for carbon dioxide removal)
• increase breath size – increase PIP or reduce PEEP.

METABOLIC ACIDOSIS
In extremely preterm infants it may be due to:
• circulatory hypoperfusion
• hypoxemia
• urinary loss of bicarbonate (alkaline urine)
• anemia
• parenteral nutrition.

High-frequency oscillatory ventilation (see Chapter 25)

Initial ventilator settings

• Mean airway pressure – 2 cm above conventional, or about 8 cm H$_2$O for preterm with respiratory distress syndrome.
• Delta pressure – 20 cm H$_2$O.
• Frequency – 10 Hz.
Perform chest X-ray after 1 hour to determine lung volume.

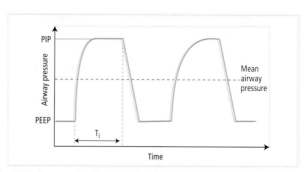

Fig. 72.3 Oxygenation is proportional to mean airway pressure. (PIP, peak inspiratory pressure; PEEP, positive end-expiratory pressure; T$_i$, inspiratory time.)

Neonatal care involves a large number of practical procedures. Each has specific advantages and risks. Training and preparation are the key to success and avoiding complications. Consider how to minimize discomfort or pain and what is the optimal time from the baby's perspective in relation to feeds and other procedures. Some common procedures are shown in Table 73.1.

Table 73.1 Some common procedures.

Procedure	Preparation and equipment	Comments	Technique	Advantages	Risks
Capillary blood sampling (heelstick)	Clean procedure Gloves, sterile alcohol swab, automatic mini-lancet, tubes, gauze	Autostylets less painful. Avoid undue squeezing of heel, as painful and gives misleading results	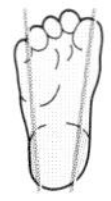 **Fig. 73.1** Shaded areas show site for capillary sampling.	Simple technique for blood glucose, hematocrit, complete blood count, electrolytes and blood gases	If results are abnormal, confirm with venipuncture Bruising Infection Rarely osteomyelitis
Venous sampling of blood	Clean procedure Gloves, sterile alcohol swab, needle, tubes for blood sample, gauze	Do not use standard needle with hub removed i.e. 'broken needle' technique Avoid potential sites for central venous access	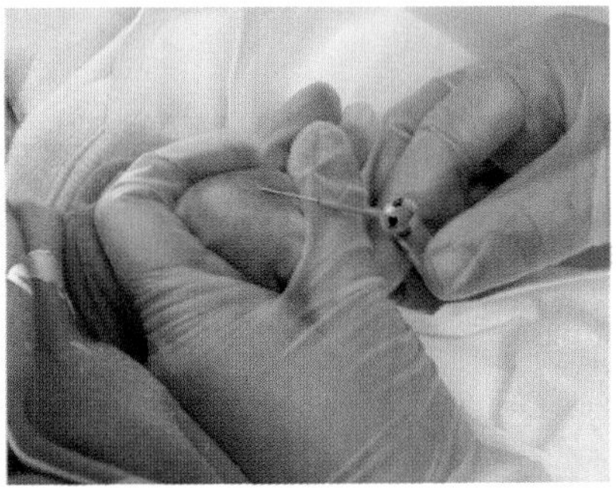 **Fig. 73.2** Venous blood sampling from back of the hand.	Good flow of blood – avoids hemolysis of sample	Bruising Infection Difficult access in some infants
Peripheral venous cannulation	Clean procedure Gloves, sterile alcohol swab, cannulae, flushed T-piece, stopper, syringe, tape, dressing	Fiber-optic light may facilitate visualization of veins Leave site of cannula tip visible to be inspected	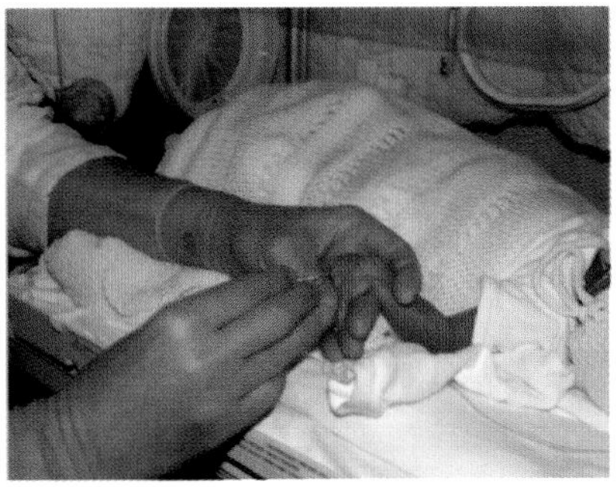 **Fig. 73.3** Peripheral venous cannulation. When blood flows back, advance cannula over needle.	Usually relatively quick access	Bruising Inflammation Infection Extravasation injury
Peripheral arterial cannulation	Clean procedure Gloves, sterile alcohol swab, cannulae, flushed T-piece, stopper, tape, dressing	Hand: radial artery Foot: posterior tibial, dorsalis pedis Do not use temporal artery Infuse heparinized saline	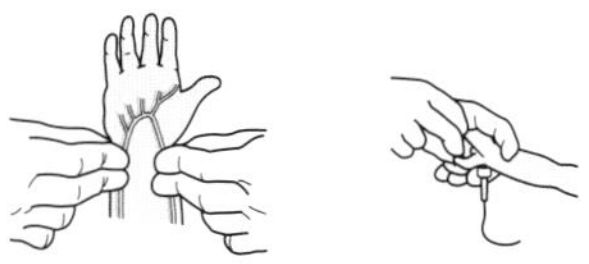 **Fig. 73.4** Peripheral arterial cannulation. (a) Check collaterals (Allen test) – hand blanches when both arteries occluded; color returns when occlusion of one artery is released. (b) Cannula insertion is facilitated by a fiber-optic light.	Access for repeated blood sampling Accurate BP measurement unless poor peripheral circulation	Blood loss if line disconnected If poor perfusion of fingers/toes – **REMOVE** Rarely ischemia or gangrene

Table 73.1 *(continued)*

Procedure	Preparation and equipment	Comments	Technique	Advantages	Risks
Urinary catheter	Sterile procedure. Gloves, sterile towel, cleaning fluid, nasogastric tubes 4 or 5 FG	To obtain sterile urine. Also for monitoring urinary output in renal failure		Simpler and more reliable in obtaining a specimen than suprapubic aspirate and no needlestick	Urethral damage Hemorrhage Contaminated urine sample
Suprapubic aspirate (bladder tap)	Clean procedure Gloves, sterile alcohol swab, needle, syringe, sterile pot, gauze	Higher success rate if ultrasound abdomen to check if bladder is full		Sterile sampling for reliable diagnosis of urinary tract infection	Rare – hemorrhage or needlestick injury to bowel
Lumbar puncture	Sterile procedure Gloves, sterile towels, cleaning fluid, gauze, LP needles, containers for CSF samples	Position infant lying on side or sitting with spine flexed. Slowly advance needle with stylet in direction of umbilicus. May feel a give when entering subarachnoid space	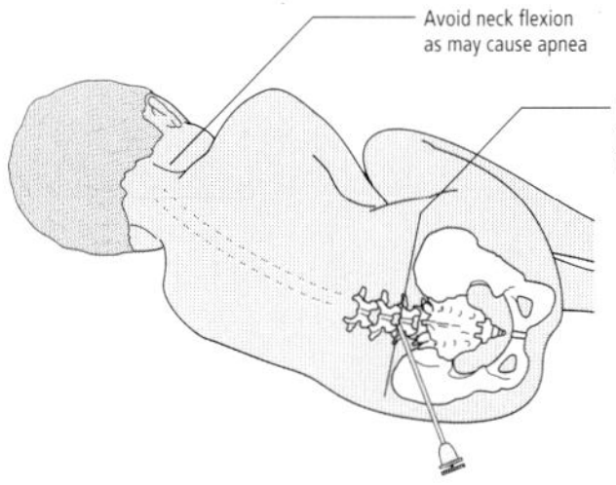 Avoid neck flexion as may cause apnea Usually L4/5 space is just below line joining iliac crests **Fig. 73.5** Lumbar puncture. Back curved, but avoid neck flexion as may cause apnea. Usually L4/5 space, i.e. just below line joining iliac crests.	Identifies meningitis Treatment of post-hemorrhagic hydrocephalus Rarely, screening for metabolic disorder	Blood-stained CSF – trauma or hemorrhage (intraventricular or subarachnoid) Contraindicated: • bleeding diathesis e.g. thrombocytopenia • cardiorespiratory instability

Umbilical catheters

Umbilical artery catheter (UAC)

Indications
- Continuous measurement of arterial blood pressure.
- Frequent blood gases and other blood samples; continuous blood gas measurement becoming available.
- Exchange transfusion – to remove blood.

Insertion
- Measure length (cord to nipple line + 9 cm to position at T10) or measure umbilicus to shoulder and use graph as Fig. 73.6.
- Prime catheter with saline.
- Sterile technique, identify artery (Fig. 73.7), insert 3 or 4.5 F gauge catheter (Fig. 73.8).

Position of catheter (Fig. 73.9)
- Low: L4–L5.
- High: T6–T10.
- Avoid tip at renal, celiac and mesenteric arteries.
- Check position with X-ray (Fig. 73.10) or ultrasound.

Management
- Secure catheter (Fig. 73.8).
- Heparinize line.
- Remove when no longer required.

Complications
- Poor perfusion of lower limbs – immediately **REMOVE**.
- May withdraw significant blood volume from sampling – keep an accurate record of volume of blood samples.
- Blood loss if line disconnects.
- Aortic thrombosis and emboli.
- Infection.

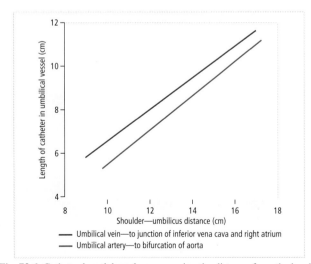

Fig. 73.6 Catheter length based on measuring the distance from the level of the distal ends of the clavicles to the umbilicus. (Adapted from Dunn P. Localization of the umbilical catheter by post-mortem measurement. *Arch Dis Child* 1966; **41**: 69.)

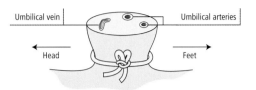

Fig. 73.7 Two arteries and one vein in umbilicus.

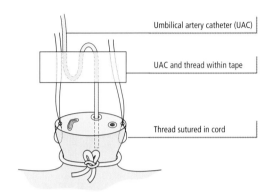

Fig. 73.8 Insertion and fixation of umbilical artery catheter. Transverse cutting of cord and dilating artery, as shown here, or cut-down onto artery. Magnification may be helpful. The umbilical cord is tied to a strip of tape to avoid tape on the skin.

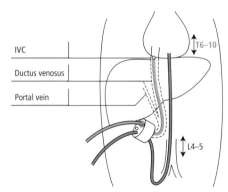

Fig. 73.9 Correct position of umbilical and venous catheters.

Umbilical vein catheter (UVC)

Indications
- Resuscitation – for intravenous access.
- Inotropes.
- Total parenteral nutrition.
- Exchange transfusion.

Insertion
- Measure length (cord to nipple line + 5 cm) for high UVC position or measure umbilicus to shoulder and use graph (Fig. 73.6).
- Sterile technique.
- Single or double lumen.
- Prime catheter with saline (or seal end if emergency use).

Position of line
- Low – 7 cm in term infants for resuscitation.
- High (preferred) – in inferior vena cava.
- Avoid tip in portal vein or opposite renal veins.
- Check position with X-ray (Fig. 73.10) or ultrasound.

Management
Remove as soon as no longer essential.

Complications
- Thrombosis or emboli.
- Hepatic damage.
- Infection.
- Pleural or pericardial effusion (if in right atrium).

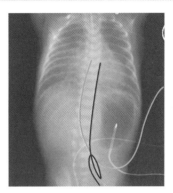

Fig. 73.10 X-ray to confirm position of the umbilical artery (red) and umbilical vein (blue) catheters, which need to be withdrawn. Also check position of tracheal tube (satisfactory) and nasogastric tube (missing).

Central venous catheters

In neonatal units, central catheters are usually peripherally inserted (PICC lines), but sometimes a surgically placed subclavian catheter is required for long-term management.

Peripherally inserted central catheters (PICC lines)

Indications
- Total parenteral nutrition – often in preterm infants or after surgery.
- Inotropes.
- Hyperosmolar infusions, e.g. glucose >12.5%.

Insertion (Figs 74.1 and 74.2)
- Prepare infant – analgesia, sedation, place in optimal position, temperature control, monitoring, measure length of line from cannulation site to inferior or superior vena cava.
- Prepare equipment – gauze, polyurethane catheter, cannula for insertion, T-piece and connection, dressing, saline flush.
- Sterile procedure – wear two sets of gloves and remove outer gloves once placement area cleaned and sterile.

Position of line
- Ideal position of the tip is in the inferior or superior vena cava just distal to but **not in** the right atrium.
- Position of the long line should be checked initially by X-ray (Fig. 74.3) and subsequently by ultrasound scans or X-ray to check not migrated to right atrium.
- If line inserted in upper arm, X-ray for position with arm abducted.

Management
- Lines usually last 10 days to 2 or more weeks.

Complications
- Infection.
- Thrombus and emboli.
- Extravasation – pleural effusion, pericardial effusion causing tamponade, tissue edema.
- Superior vena caval obstruction.
- Blockage.
- Leakage at connection sites.
- Line breaking off on removal.

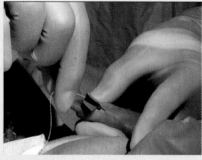

Fig. 74.1 Insertion of cannula. The long line is threaded through the cannula. Non-toothed forceps may be used.

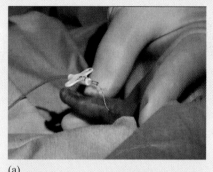

(a)

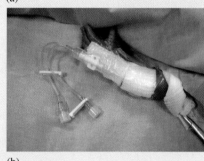

(b)

Fig. 74.2 (a) Central catheter in place. (b) Dressing with infusion site visible. Infant comfortable, dressing not constricting, easy to redress if required.

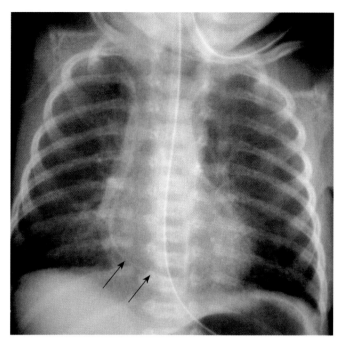

Fig. 74.3 X-ray demonstrating importance of confirming catheter position. The central venous catheter is in the right atrium (arrows) and must be withdrawn.

Subclavian

Indications
- Long-term central access.
- Peripheral insertion not possible.

Insertion
- Usually by a pediatric surgeon or interventional radiologist under general anesthetic in operating theater.
- Tunneled under skin.

Position
- Superior vena cava.

Complications
- Pneumothorax.
- Surgical scar.
- Superior vena caval obstruction.
- Blockage.
- Infection.

Intraosseous cannulation

Indication
- Emergency infusion of fluids and medications and no venous access possible (not sodium bicarbonate).

Preparation
- Sterile procedure.
- Position infant with knee flexed and supported.

Sites of insertion
- Proximal tibia 1–3 cm below tibial tuberosity – medial flat surface (Fig. 74.4)
- Insert needle at 10–15 degrees towards foot (avoids growth plate).
- Use twisting motion.
- Dressing.

Complications
- Fracture.
- Cellulitis/osteomyelitis.

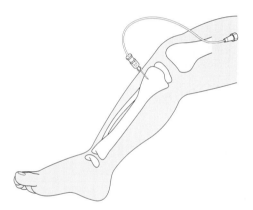

Fig. 74.4 Intraosseous infusion in tibia.

Chest tubes

Indications

- Pneumothorax.
- Pleural effusion.

Technique

- Sites:
  - lateral – 3rd to 5th intercostal space, anterior axillary line
  - anterior – 3rd intercostal space, mid-clavicular line.
- Avoid nipple and breast bud.
- Aseptic technique.
- Approach – upper edge of rib.
- Local anesthesia – 1% lidocaine (lignocaine) and intravenous analgesia.
- Small incision along skin line. Blunt dissection of intercostal muscle with forceps.
- Use either an 8FG or 10FG chest tube or a pigtail catheter.
- Insert without trocar to reduce risk of damaging lung.
- Connect tube to valve or underwater seal, observe air bubbles and swinging with respiration.
- Fix the tube to chest wall with Tegaderm and Steristrips or a suture.
- X-ray to check tube position and lung re-expansion (Fig. 75.1).

Complications

- Hemothorax.
- Surgical emphysema.
- Scarring of skin or breast tissue.

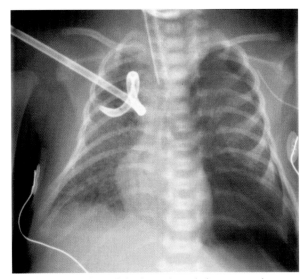

Fig. 75.1 X-ray showing a right chest tube to drain a pneumothorax. Pulmonary interstitial emphysema (PIE) is present in the right lung. There is a left pneumothorax with lung collapse and mediastinal shift to the right.

Pleural tap

Indications

- Pleural fluid.

Technique

- Aseptic.
- Ultrasound-guided to identify fluid.
- Local anesthesia – 1% lidocaine (lignocaine) and intravenous analgesia.
- Small incision along skin line. Blunt dissection of intercostal muscle with forceps.
- Insert a 22G cannula just above the rib.
- Attach to three-way tap.
- Aspirate fluid with a syringe.

Complications

- Pneumothorax.
- Hemothorax.

Chest needling

Indication

- Tension pneumothorax – if immediate treatment is required.

Technique

- Site – 2nd or 3rd intercostal space, mid-clavicular line.
- Insert cannula. Create underwater seal.
- Usually followed by chest tube insertion.

Exchange transfusion

Indications

- Severe unconjugated hyperbilirubinemia – exchange with fresh blood (CMV-negative), 2 × blood volume.
- Polycythemia – exchange with normal saline, to reduce hematocrit to 0.55 (approx. 20 ml/kg).

Technique

Via peripheral venous and peripheral or umbilical arterial lines
- Infuse blood at a constant rate through the vein via a blood warmer.
- Withdraw blood from arterial line in aliquots (5–10 ml).

Via umbilical venous catheter
- Alternate between withdrawing and infusing aliquots (5–10 ml) of blood.

Monitoring

- Vital signs throughout.
- Volume infused and withdrawn.
- Allow time for equilibration – perform over 1 hour for double volume exchange.

Complications

- Technical problems.
- Air embolization or thrombosis.
- Volume overload or depletion.
- Electrolyte imbalance – hyperkalemia, hypocalcemia, acidosis or alkalosis (check before, during and afterwards).
- Hypoglycemia.
- Infection.
- Hypothermia.
- Mortality – possibly up to 1%.

The anterior fontanel provides an ideal window for obtaining cranial ultrasound images. Ultrasound is especially helpful in identifying brain injury in preterm infants. The examination is non-invasive and can be performed at the bedside with minimal disturbance to the infant. Serial imaging allows monitoring of progression or resolution of lesions, which is much more informative than an individual scan.

Ultrasound images of the brain vary with gestational and postnatal age. At early gestation, the cortex is relatively smooth with few cerebral fissures, sulci and gyri. By term, the surface of the cortex appears convoluted and sulci and gyral patterns are well developed.

Indications

- Infants < 1500 g birthweight or < 32 weeks' gestation.
- Infants requiring intensive care.
- Neurologic abnormality – clinical, seizures, encephalopathy.
- Antenatally detected abnormality.

Lesions that can be identified

Preterm infants

- Hemorrhage.
- Ventricular dilatation.
- Periventricular leukomalacia.

All infants

- Range of CNS congenital abnormalities.
- Ventricular dilatation.
- Cerebral edema.
- Calcification from congenital infection.

Standard views for scans

Coronal views (Fig. 76.1)

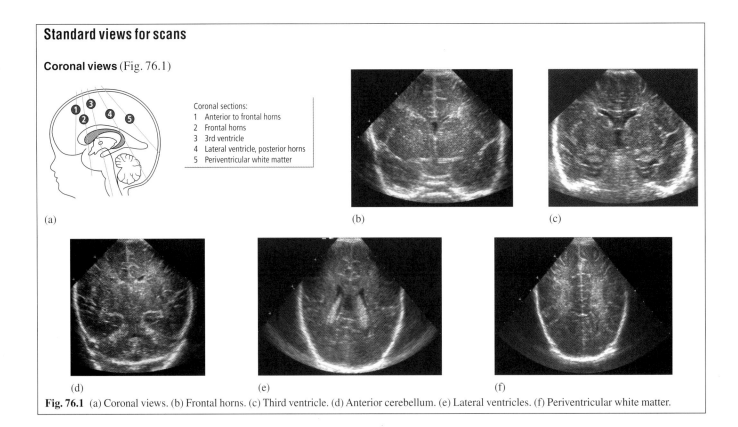

Coronal sections:
1 Anterior to frontal horns
2 Frontal horns
3 3rd ventricle
4 Lateral ventricle, posterior horns
5 Periventricular white matter

(a)　　(b)　　(c)

(d)　　(e)　　(f)

Fig. 76.1 (a) Coronal views. (b) Frontal horns. (c) Third ventricle. (d) Anterior cerebellum. (e) Lateral ventricles. (f) Periventricular white matter.

Sagittal views (Fig. 76.2)

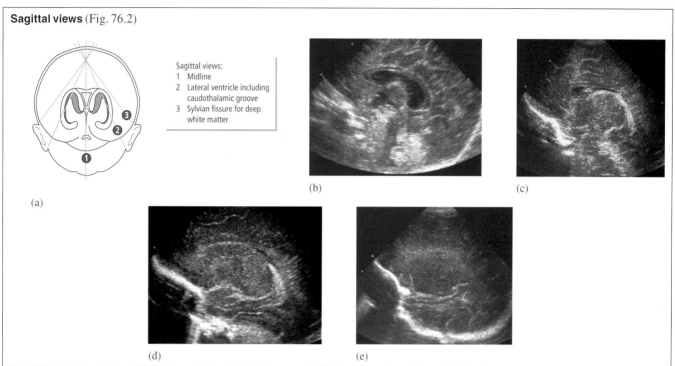

Sagittal views:
1 Midline
2 Lateral ventricle including caudothalamic groove
3 Sylvian fissure for deep white matter

(a)

(b)

(c)

(d)

(e)

Fig. 76.2 (a) Sagittal views. (b) Midline. (c) Caudothalamic groove. (d) Body of lateral ventricle. (e) Sylvian fissure.

Hemorrhage, ventricular dilatation

Germinal matrix hemorrhage (Grade 1) (Fig. 76.3)

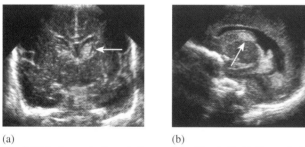

(a)

(b)

Fig. 76.3 Left germinal matrix hemorrhage (Grade 1). (a) Coronal view. (b) Sagittal view.

Intraventricular hemorrhage (Grade 2 – no ventricular dilatation) (Fig. 76.4)

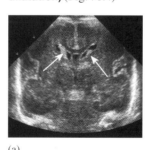

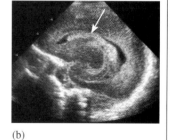

(a)

(b)

Fig. 76.4 Bilateral intraventricular hemorrhage (Grade 2). (a) Coronal view. (b) Sagittal view.

(continued)

Intraventricular hemorrhage (Grade 3 – ventricular dilatation) (Fig. 76.5)

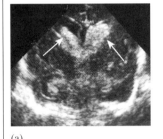
(a)

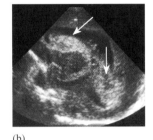
(b)

Fig. 76.5 Bilateral intraventricular hemorrhage (Grade 3). (a) Coronal view. (b) Sagittal view.

Hemorrhagic parenchymal infarct (Grade 4) (Fig. 76.6)

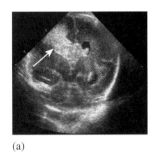
(a)

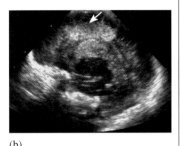
(b)

Fig. 76.6 Right hemorrhagic parenchymal infarct (Grade 4). (a) Coronal view. (b) Sagittal view.

Ventricular dilatation (Figs 76.7–9)

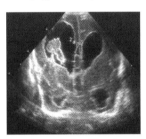

Fig. 76.7 Marked bilateral ventricular dilatation and hemorrhage in right ventricle on coronal scan.

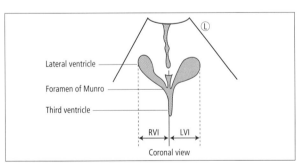

Fig. 76.8 Ventricular index, measured from the midline to the lateral border of the ventricle on a coronal scan in the plane of the third ventricle. Other indices can be used. (LVI, left ventricular index; RVI, right ventricular index.)

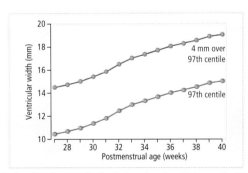

Fig. 76.9 Centiles for ventricular index showing 97th centile. The upper line is when treatment is likely to be required. (Levene MI, *Arch Dis Child* 1981; **56**: 900–904.)

Periventricular leukomalacia (PVL) (Figs 75.10 and 75.11)

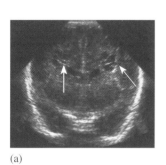

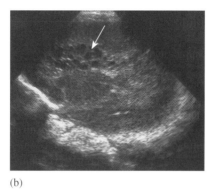

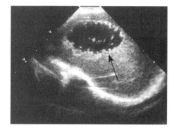

(a)   (b)

Fig. 76.10 Widespread subcortical cysts on day 55 in (a) coronal and (b) sagittal views. Initial scans are normal or show increased periventricular echogenicity.

Fig. 76.11 Porencephalic cyst at site of a unilateral hemorrhagic parenchymal infarct.

Limitations of ultrasound

- Cannot reliably distinguish between hemorrhage and infarction.
- Poor sensitivity in identifying:
  - cerebral white matter injury in preterm or after hypoxic-ischemic encephalopathy
  - cerebral edema
  - subdural, subgaleal (subaponeurotic) hemorrhage.

MRI imaging is more sensitive in identifying these lesions.

Practical issues

- Always clean the probe before and after use with each infant.
- Record images.
- Never report an abnormality unless visible on both coronal and sagittal views.
- Enter written report by experienced neonatologist or radiologist into patient record.

Question

When can the lesions in VLBW infants be identified?

Shortly after birth – identifies antenatal and early injury – small cysts, flares, hemorrhage.

During first week – hemorrhage, early ventricular dilatation, flares.

Next few weeks – ventricular dilatation, cysts from PVL and if lesions progress or resolve.

At discharge or term – most useful for prognosis, but reliability is limited.

Neonatologists are increasingly using echocardiography to assist with the immediate management of the acutely ill infant, to:
- identify and evaluate shunting across a patent ductus arteriosus
- assess cardiac function to determine the need and efficacy of inotropes and volume support
- identify the position of umbilical and central venous lines
- exclude major cardiac defects
- identify pulmonary hypertension
- exclude pericardial effusion.

The neonatologist should work in close collaboration with a pediatric cardiac center. When not on-site, this is increasingly achieved by using telemedicine for review of ultrasound images. However, echocardiography of complex congenital heart disease is the realm of the pediatric cardiologist or trained ultrasonographer.

Views

The standard views (Figs 77.1 and 77.2) in a neonate are:
- four-chamber
- parasternal short-axis
- parasternal long-axis
- subcostal.

High-quality images must be obtained.

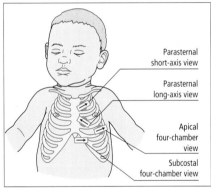

Fig. 77.1 Positions of probe and views obtained.

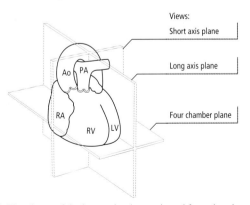

Fig. 77.2 The planes of the long axis, short axis and four-chamber apical or subcostal views.

Question

What are the different types of ultrasound imaging used in echocardiography?

With ultrasound, high-frequency (ultrasound) waves are reflected or scattered from underlying tissues. Waves of high frequency (>7.5 MHz) provide a high-resolution picture. Waves of a lower frequency penetrate to a greater tissue depth.
- **2D images** – used to ascertain cardiac anatomy; best when ultrasound waves are at right angles to target.
- **Doppler** – measures velocity of moving target (usually blood cells). Most accurate when ultrasound beam is parallel to the direction of motion of the target.
- **Color Doppler** – by convention, red indicates flow towards the probe and blue away. Turbulent flow produces variable colors.
- **Pulsed wave Doppler** – bursts of ultrasound from a focal point. A smooth recording indicates non-turbulent flow.
- **Continuous wave Doppler** – receives information from whole field; used when high-flow velocity is suspected.
- **M mode** – displays cross-sectional images of the heart.

Four-chamber view

- Confirms (Figs 77.3 and 77.4):
  - there are four chambers – appropriate size
  - there are normal mitral and tricuspid valves, and tricuspid is offset, i.e. lower
  - ventricular septum intact.
- Quantifies the degree of tricuspid regurgitation – useful for estimating pulmonary artery pressure.

Short-axis view

This view (Figs 77.5 and 77.6) allows identification of:
- patent ductus arteriosus
- perimembranous ventricular septal defect (VSD)
- usual arrangement of pulmonary artery and aorta
- structural defects, e.g. transposition of the great arteries, pulmonary stenosis.

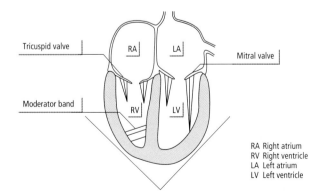

Fig. 77.3 Four-chamber view. The right ventricle can be identified from a band of tissue, the moderator band.

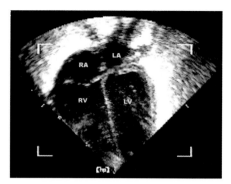

Fig. 77.4 Ultrasound showing four-chamber view.

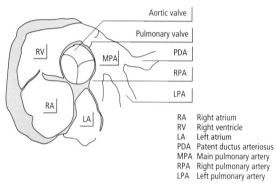

RA   Right atrium
RV   Right ventricle
LA   Left atrium
PDA   Patent ductus arteriosus
MPA   Main pulmonary artery
RPA   Right pulmonary artery
LPA   Left pulmonary artery

Fig. 77.5 Short-axis view.

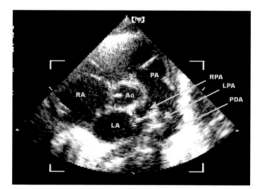

Fig. 77.6 Ultrasound of short-axis view.

Long-axis view

This view (Figs 77.7 and 77.8) is used to:
- identify correct position of pulmonary artery and aorta
- detect structural defects, e.g. tetralogy of Fallot
- assess volume overload in a patent ductus arteriosus (left atrial: aortic root ratio).

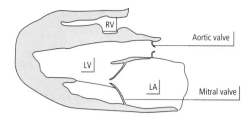

RV   Right ventricle
LA   Left atrium
LV   Left ventricle

Fig. 77.7 Long-axis view.

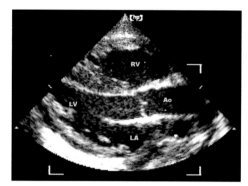

Fig. 77.8 Ultrasound showing long-axis view.

Subcostal view

This view is used to:
- check liver on right and aorta on left side, i.e. situs solitus
- obtain high-quality images if other views affected by lung hyperinflation or high-frequency oscillation (HFOV)
- check position of central lines in inferior vena cava or aorta.

Patent ductus arteriosus

See Chapter 32.

Assessment of left ventricular function in critically ill neonates

Is there poor cardiac contractility or volume depletion? Echocardiography allows subjective assessment of cardiac contractility from the variation in left ventricle size. Left ventricular shortening fraction can be used to estimate systolic function. Assessment of cardiac volume loading is more difficult, particularly in the first few days of life, with the added complexity of the transitional circulation. On the subcostal view, inferior vena caval filling can be observed as a guide to intravascular volume – it is collapsed with hypovolemia. Three-dimensional echocardiography and reconstructive magnetic resonance imaging are being developed to quantify cardiac chamber size and provide more accurate functional assessments.

Gestational age assessment: Ballard exam

Gestational age can be assessed clinically (±2 weeks) from the changes in neuromuscular and physical maturity with gestation. The most widely used scoring systems are the Dubowitz and the somewhat shorter Ballard score shown in Fig. 78.1 and Table 78.1.

Maturity rating

Add up the individual neuromuscular and physical maturity scores for the 12 categories, then obtain the estimated gestational age from Table 78.2. The neuromuscular maturity score may be unreliable if the infant is sedated or ill.

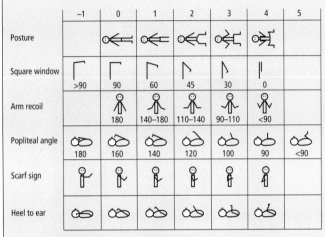

Fig. 78.1 Neuromuscular maturity.

Table 78.2 Gestational age estimated from summed neuromuscular and physical maturity scores.

Total score	Gestational age (weeks)
−10	20
−5	22
0	24
5	26
10	28
15	30
20	32
25	34
30	36
35	38
40	40
45	42
50	44

Table 78.1 Physical maturity scores.

Sign	−1	0	1	2	3	4	5
Skin	Sticky, friable, transparent	Gelatinous red, translucent	Smooth pink, visible veins	Superficial peeling and/or rash, few veins	Cracking, pale areas, rare veins	Parchment, deep cracking, no vessels	Leathery, cracked, wrinkled
Lanugo	None	Sparse	Abundant	Thinning	Bald areas	Mostly bald	
Plantar creases	Heel–toe 40–50 mm = −1 <40 mm = −2	Heel–toe >50 mm, no creases	Faint red marks	Anterior transverse crease only	Creases over anterior 2/3	Creases over entire sole	
Breast	Imperceptible	Barely perceptible	Flat areola, no bud	Stippled areola, bud 1–2 mm	Raised areola, bud 3–4 mm	Full areola, bud 5–10 mm	
Eye and ear	Lids fused loosely = −1, tightly = −2	Lids open, pinna flat, stays folded	Slightly curved pinna, soft with slow recoil	Well-curved pinna, soft but ready recoil	Formed and firm, with instant recoil	Thick cartilage, ear stiff	
Genitalia, male	Scrotum flat, smooth	Scrotum empty, faint rugae	Testes in upper canal, rare rugae	Testes descending, few rugae	Testes down, good rugae	Testes pendulous, deep rugae	
Genitalia, female	Clitoris prominent, labia flat	Prominent clitoris, small labia minora	Prominent clitoris, enlarging minora	Majora and minora equally prominent	Majora large, minora small	Majora cover clitoris and minora	

Blood pressure charts (Figs 78.2 and 78.3)

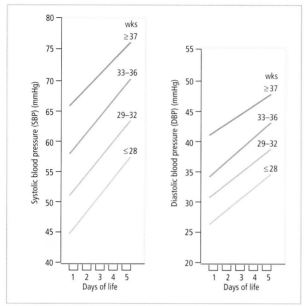

Fig. 78.2 Systolic and diastolic blood pressure by age and gestational age. (From Zubrow AB *et al*. Determinants of blood pressure in infants admitted to neonatal intensive care units: A prospective multicenter study. Philadelphia Neonatal Blood Pressure Study Group. *J Perinatol* 1995; **15**: 470.)

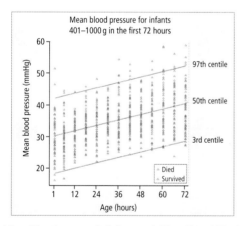

Fig. 78.3 Mean blood pressure in infants weighing 401–1000 g in first 72 hours of life. (Courtesy of Dr Jon Fanaroff, 2003.)

Severity of illness scores

Used to adjust outcomes according to severity of illness. The most widely used in neonatology are:
- SNAP-PE II score
- CRIB II score.

The SNAP-PE II (Score Neonatal Acute Physiology Perinatal Extension) is based on the physiologic derangement in a number of organ systems (urine output, mean blood pressure, worst PaO_2/FiO_2 ratio, lowest serum pH, occurrence of seizures) in the first 12 hours after admission to the NICU (neonatal intensive care unit), birth weight, Apgar score at 5 minutes, and whether there is IUGR (intra-uterine growth restriction).

The CRIB (Clinical Risk Index for Babies) score is for very low birthweight (VLBW) infants and is based on birth weight, gestation, maximal base excess, in the first 12 hours of life and temperature on admission.

The use of the SNAP-PE is limited by the complexity of the data required and the CRIB score by the overwhelming effects of birth weight and gestational age on outcome.

Index